KILTED YOGA

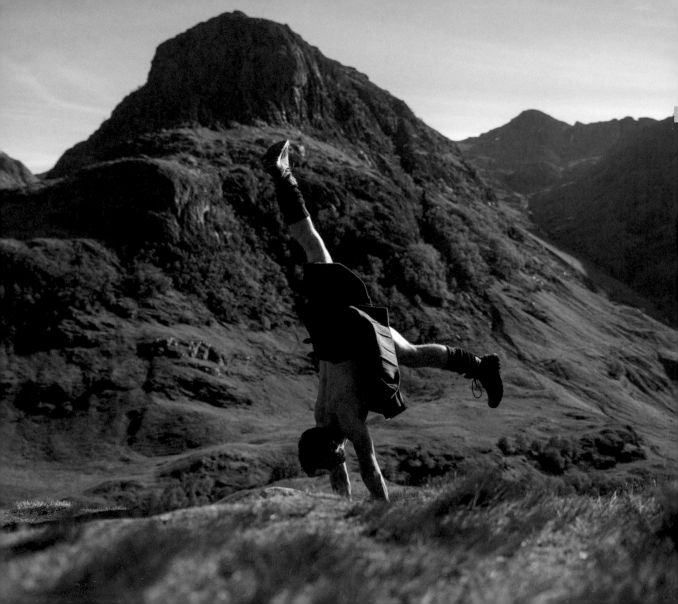

KILTED YOGA

YOGA LAID BARE

FINLAY WILSON

First published in Great Britain in 2017 by Yellow Kite
An imprint of Hodder & Stoughton
An Hachette UK company

3

A CIP catalogue record for this title is available from the British Library

Hardback ISBN 978 1 473 66784 6
eBook ISBN 978 1 473 66785 3

Colour origination by Born Group
Printed and bound in Italy by L.E.G.O Spa

Hodder & Stoughton policy is to use papers that are natural, renewable and recyclable
products and made from wood grown in sustainable forests. The logging and
manufacturing processes are expected to conform to the environmental regulations
of the country of origin.

Yellow Kite
Hodder & Stoughton Ltd
Carmelite House
50 Victoria Embankment
London EC4Y 0DZ

www.yellowkitebooks.co.uk
www.hodder.co.uk

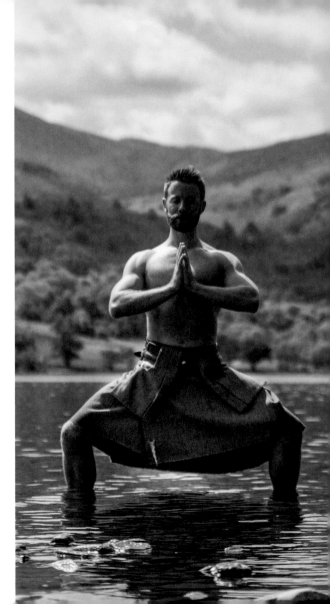

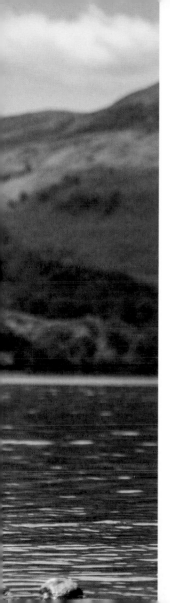

CONTENTS

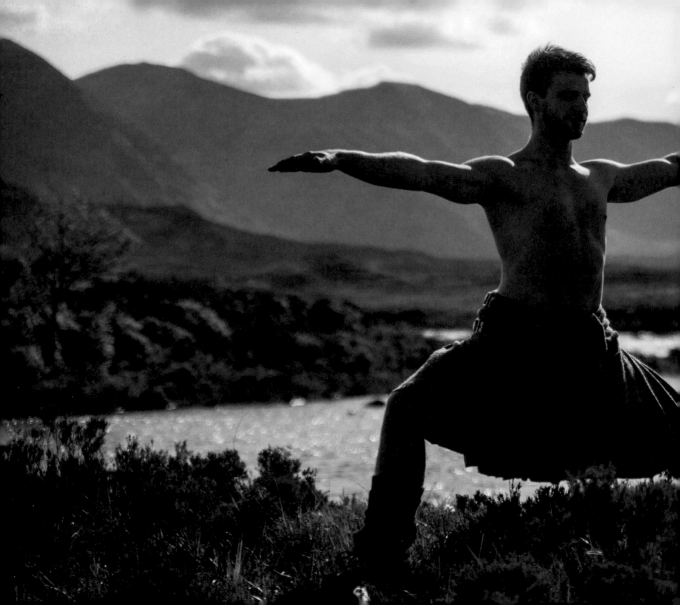

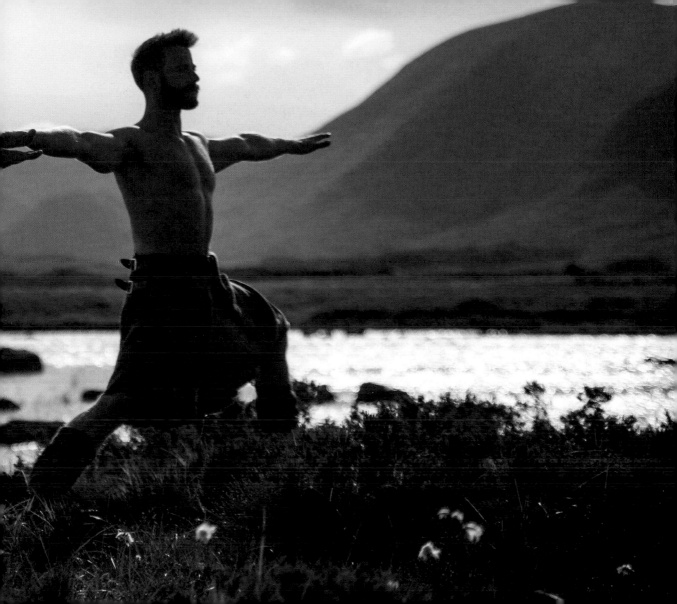

INTRODUCTION

THE STORY BEHIND KILTED YOGA

In 2016 I was asked to become a contributor to BBC The Social, an online platform that features creative people across Scotland. I wanted to bring my sense of humour to the content and so I proposed a video of yoga in kilts, shot in the style of an aftershave commercial. In fact, this idea wasn't their first choice. It wasn't until my rescue dog, Amaloh, went viral with 2.6 million views that I was encouraged to create the Kilted Yoga video.

Kilts in hand, Tristan and I went to the Hermitage in Perthshire; it reminded me of where I grew up and its setting encapsulates features of the Scottish landscape. We were freezing the whole time, especially when shooting that final 'cheeky' headstand at the end! After Tristan fell out of the headstand for the 50th time, I had to call time on the shoot as I could no longer feel my hands or feet, and snow was starting to fall all around us.

The afternoon the video went out I was due to be teaching. After my first one-hour class, I saw that we had passed 1 million views. After the second class, I was shocked to see that we now had 2 million views. By the next morning we had hit 17 million and I called Tristan, shaking and yelling! We couldn't believe it. It was surfacing all over the globe as people shared this 48-second video.

Articles appeared in *Cosmopolitan*, *People*, *The New York Times*, Mashable and Insider, and the story was picked up by news stations all over the world. While waiting in the BBC green room for an interview, we were speaking live to news channels in Australia. This culminated in us representing Visit Scotland on the Tartan Day Parade in New York, doing yoga down Sixth Avenue to cheering crowds and taking more than 300 selfies with fans. It has been an absolute roller coaster!

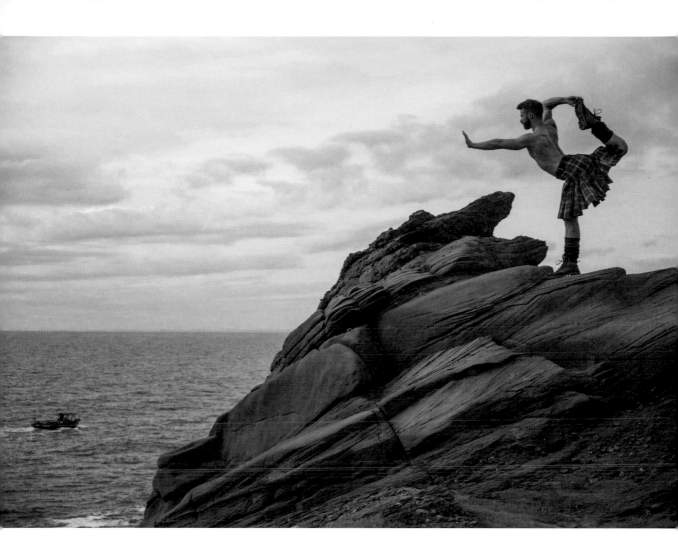

WHO IS THIS BOOK FOR?

This book is for everybody. You don't need to be a guy; you
don't even need to own a kilt! The poses and sequences will
guide you through the basics towards a stronger practice and
offer a balance of forward bends, twists and backbends to help
you strengthen and open your body in a comprehensive way.
Whether you are new to yoga or an experienced practitioner, you
can approach the poses in a new way and deepen your practice.

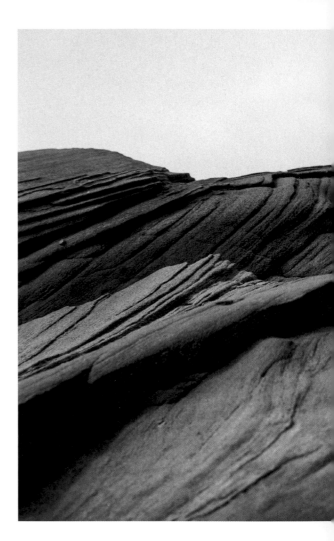

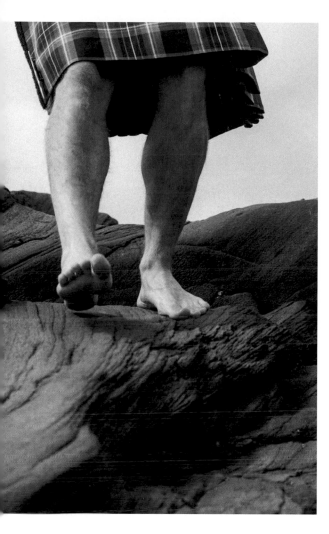

HOW TO USE THIS BOOK

This book contains four sequences to take you through the
absolute basics, building the foundations and your understanding
for the longer sequences. Each sequence builds on the one before.
There are also short meditation exercises that you can use, and
even record and play back for yourself. The meditation segments
advise on whether you should practise them alone or get out into
nature. Like any muscle, your focus needs to be regularly flexed.
The meditation examples will sharpen your attention and help
calm your mind using simple techniques.

Each sequence begins with an intent for you to use
throughout the practice to build focus and guide your attention.
From there, the breathing exercises will get you breathing
consciously, helping to develop a strong focus for the poses.

The pose instructions indicate the duration they should be
held for and how many rounds should be done, and pointers are
given for when you're in them. Repeat one-sided poses on the
other side unless the poses are marked as a sequence. At the end
of each sequence, take a few minutes for intentional rest.

MY JOURNEY INTO YOGA

My introduction to yoga was challenging. I hated it when I began: I was so stiff, the poses demanded so much of me physically and mentally, and I felt unsupported by the instructor. I was fresh out of two rounds of surgery on both my legs, having had six months between operations. So, when one leg was getting better, it was the other one's turn. The operations were to remove spikes from my bones and to mend the damage to the soft tissue. The resulting nerve damage made me look like a baby deer trying to walk.

I was on mobility supports when I showed up to my first yoga class and I couldn't do any of the standing work. I attended classes for a year and found that my stamina wasn't good. I started doing short sequences at home from audio files (back before YouTube was a thing). I progressed and by the end of that year was doing two rounds of 20 minutes a day, and I began to trust my legs again. It took about five years before I felt any real competency with the basic physical poses. To this day, my left leg can still buckle if I am exhausted. One thing I will say about

myself: I am stubborn! I never gave up despite walking out of a few classes or being told to leave because of my swearing!

Now, I do yoga every day. Without it, my muscles are tight, I feel groggy and I am usually pretty snarly. Without yoga, you wouldn't want to know me! Yoga gives me time to do a daily reset, to focus on my breath and to move, sweat and reaffirm my connection to my strength.

I teach beginners primarily and usually advise that people practise yoga a few times a week initially to get a grip with the techniques and really focus on it. After a few weeks, I advise factoring back in other activities and movement styles (running, cycling, martial arts and so on) so you can see the great boost your yoga practice can bring to them. It is down to personal preference when you do your practice. For me, I practise in the morning because of a busy work schedule but my body prefers an evening practice once I have been up and about for a while.

FORREST YOGA

My practice is steady: there are some faster moments to get warmed up (Sun Salutations are great for that) and other sequences where you are holding poses a little longer than in some other styles of flow yoga. Each day, I choose a focus and build my sequence around that, taking the time to warm up fully and aiming towards an apex pose. Forrest Yoga is so adaptable that no matter what kind of day I am having, there is something I can do.

Forrest Yoga isn't about doing yoga in the woods (note the double "r") despite what the Kilted Yoga video showed! Not to say that you can't, but some days you just need to get on your yoga mat indoors. Forrest Yoga is a system of yoga that uses intelligent sequences to address the needs of the modern-day person who may be working with issues in the neck, shoulders, lower back and hips, and to work in a way that strengthens the main postural muscles, aligns the bones and creates a feeling of space. Created by Ana Forrest, my teacher, Forrest Yoga continues to be a practice that I use for my own back and hip pain following surgery and injuries sustained about ten years ago. The focus on breath, intent, strength

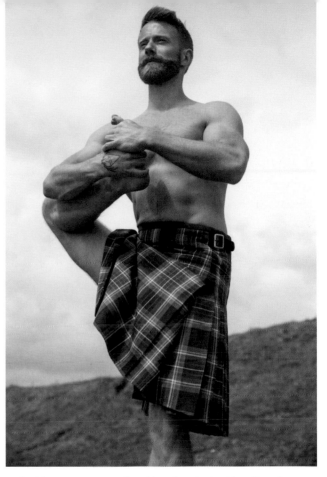

and spirit gave me a way of working that changed how I used my body and how I worked with my perception of my body and life, something that had been missing from my yoga for years.

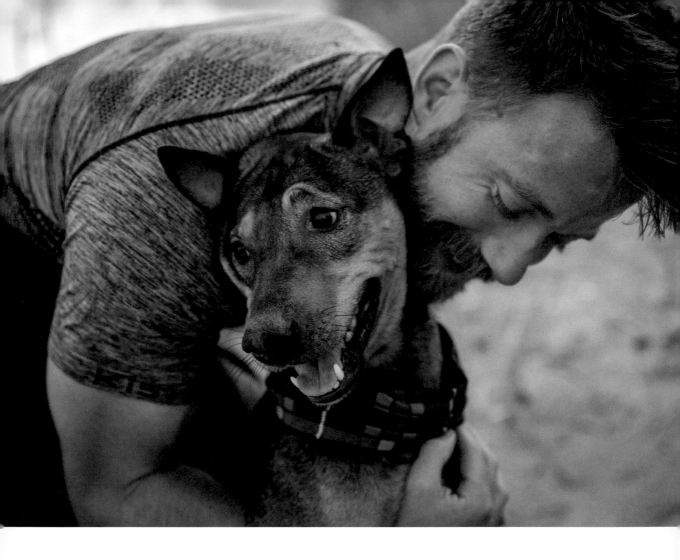

TEACHING YOGA

I began teaching yoga in Lanark, my hometown. My first classes were for adults in full-time care with multiple disabilities. After my time struggling with my body, I felt that one of my gifts was the way I could adapt poses for everyone.

When I moved north to Dundee I began teaching community classes in a few gyms around the city and thought I was really busy with three people in my class. This inspired me to open a dedicated space, something that Dundee didn't have. While looking for small properties, I stumbled upon an old church which was to be demolished and turned into flats. My then partner and I took on a huge project to turn it into an amazing space for yoga and Heart Space Yoga & Bodyworks was born. I welcomed people with disabilities to my classes and began a programme of free classes for children, teenagers and families with additional support needs; the community grew and Heart Space became my teaching base.

Now I teach all over the world while managing the studio in Dundee and I am delighted to have ten home-grown teachers alongside me who started their yoga journey with us about seven years ago. Dundee is my home and Heart Space will continue to be where I do the work I am passionate about.

LIFE GROWING UP IN RURAL SCOTLAND

I grew up on the edge of Lanark, surrounded by fields, valleys and hills for me and my three brothers to roll around in. From as young as I can remember, we were tossed out the front door and off we went to explore up the trees, in the fields of grasses taller than us and in the valley. Nature was something we had around us every day, something that I didn't realise was so important until I went to the city.

Most weekends, my dad, who is an avid mountaineer, would take us on walks locally, or on greater adventures that could take all weekend. We slept in shelters we had made ourselves, in hedges, in bothies with gas lighting and in tiny tents all over Scotland. I grew up knowing about plants and animals. I was raised in how to walk with respect in the natural world, to be quiet so we wouldn't disturb the wildlife, to conserve energy when climbing, and I learnt the rich history of the land.

Looking back, I value those times, as they created the man I am today. When I was a little older, my twin and I joined the Scouts. We soon became group leaders and developed our outdoor skills with map reading, map creation and survival skills. I went on so many adventures with friends at the weekends, in bogs with water up to my waist, in tents with ice on the inside and canoeing across lochs in the north of Scotland. Nature and the outdoors, particularly the Scottish environs, have played a big part in my life and upbringing.

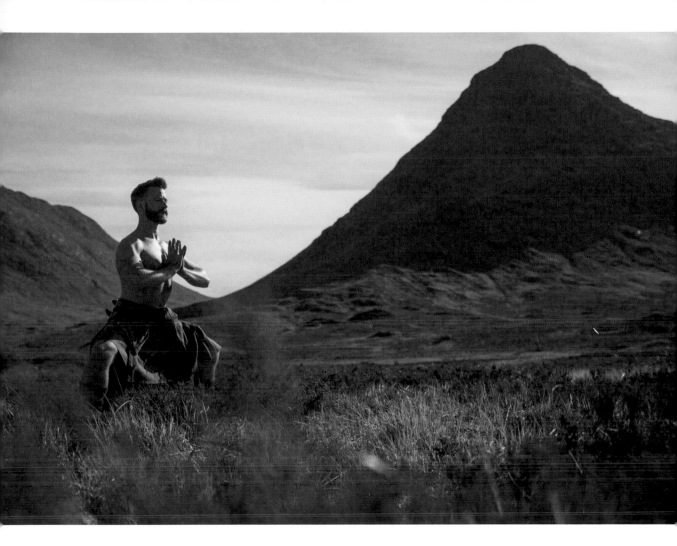

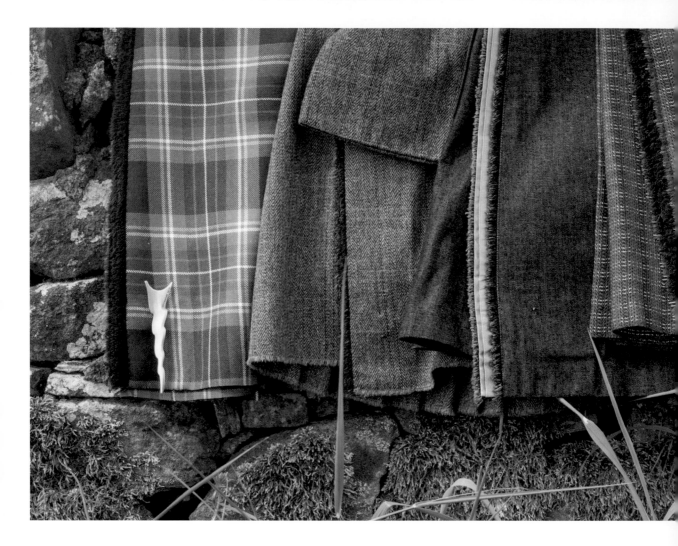

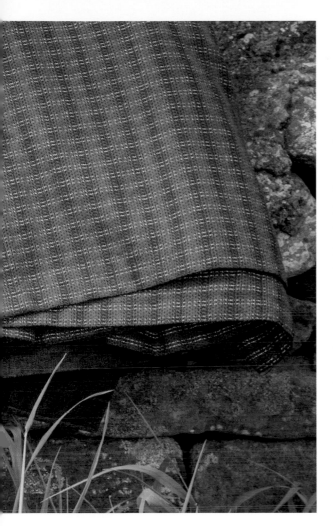

THE IMPORTANCE OF KILTS

Kilts and tartan have always been present in my life, but in
a very ceremonial way. Special occasions called for a kilt and
jacket, and for smaller events we would wear a tartan scarf
with our clan tartan. In many ways, the kilt was a subtle
presence growing up but it wasn't until I was in my late teens
that I owned my own tartan kilt and plaid. It is this kilt, with
a design called Heartland – which commemorates St Andrews
and the Kingdom of Fife where I studied – that I wore in the
Kilted Yoga video. Ten years on, that kilt has been all over the
world and worn to commemorate my heritage. For me, kilts are
a piece of heritage that reaches from the past to the present, and
I have taken to wearing them more and more, even having kilts
made with pockets to give them a modern and practical feel.

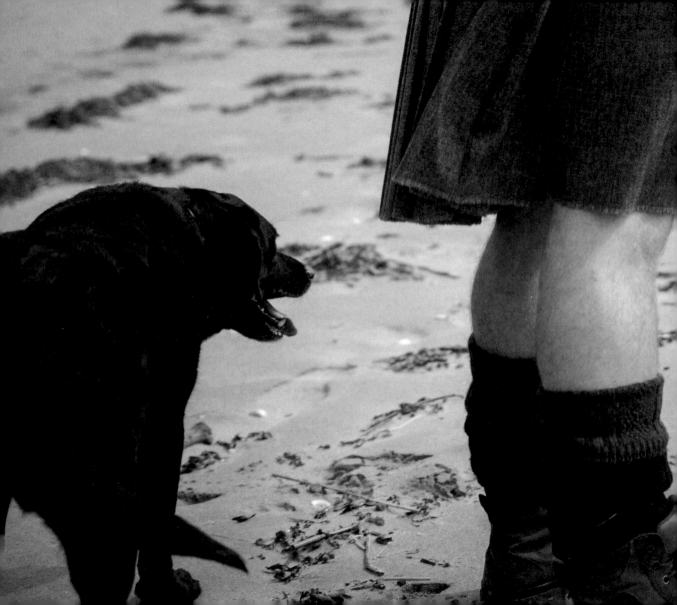

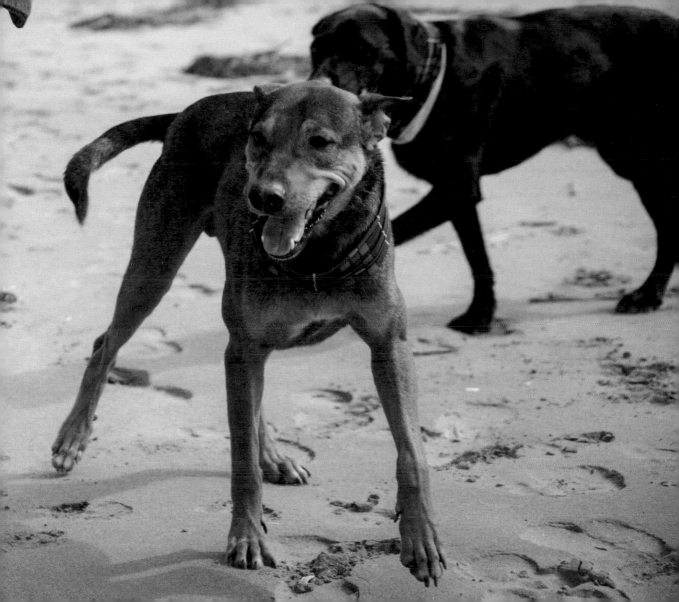

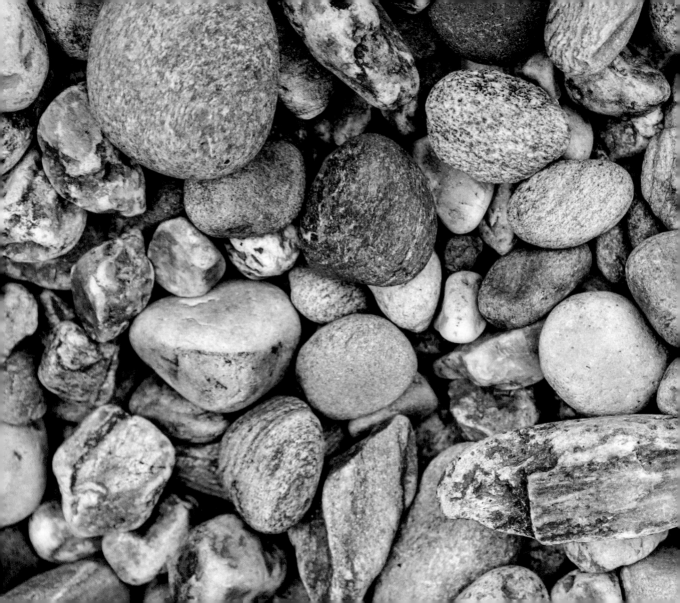

CONNECTION

INTENT: TO GRADUALLY EXPAND THE BREATH

CONNECTION

Getting focused is one of the main aims of a yoga practice and, like any skill, it requires patience and persistence. This sequence will teach you the basic moves of the practice to help set a good foundation. The poses are great to review, whether you have developed your yoga practice or are starting out. As you move through the sequence, track how deep a breath you can take and feel for when you can deepen it.

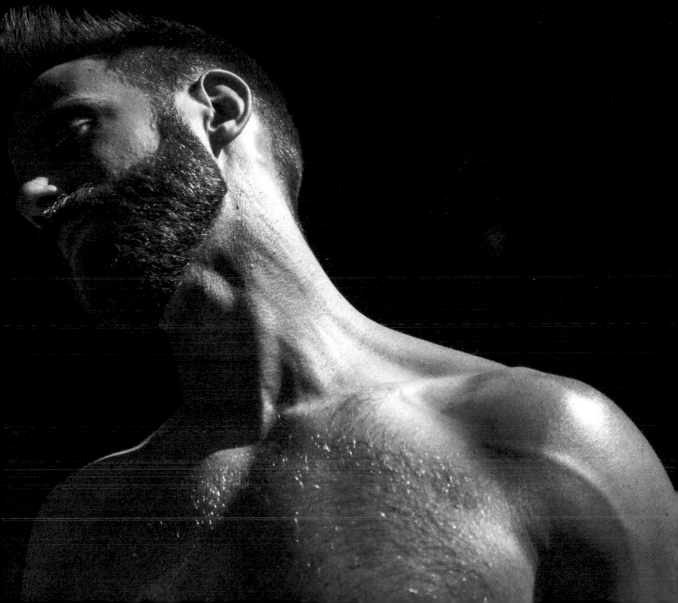

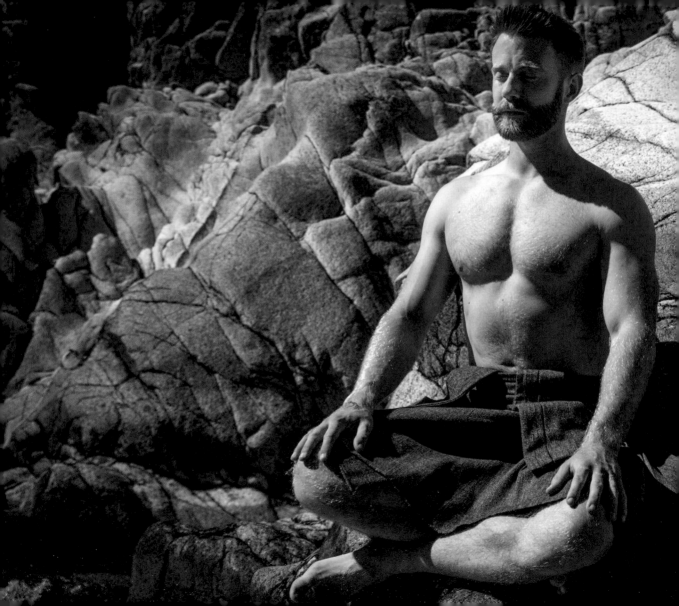

UJJAYI BREATHING

Switch to breathing in and out through the nose only. Engage the muscles in your throat that you use when whispering to add an audible quality to your breathing. Breathe steadily with this whispering sound, making the inhale and exhale even in length. (You should sound like Darth Vader.)

Ujjayi breathing should be used in all the poses except for Savasana, when you are at rest.

ACTIVE HANDS

Spread the fingers wide and feel the spread in the palms of the hands.

ACTIVE FEET

Lift and spread the toes, big toe away from pinky toe, spreading the weight evenly. Feel the engagement of the lower legs.

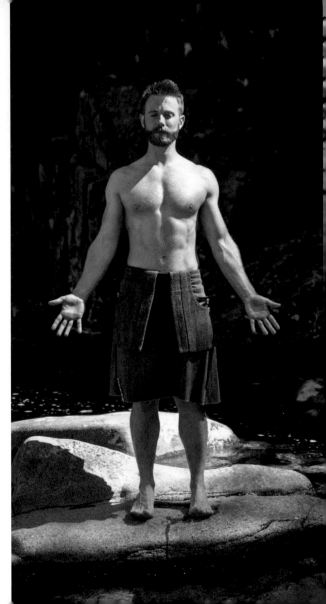

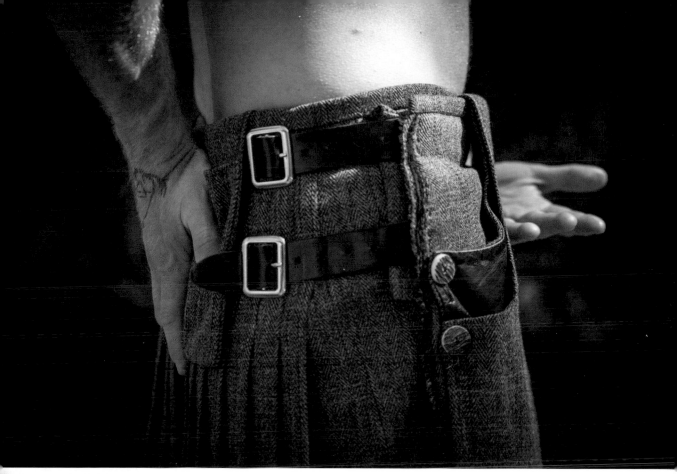

TUCKED TAIL BONE

Take one hand to tail bone and one to pubic bone. Exhale and
tuck the tail bone down to engage your lower buttock muscles.

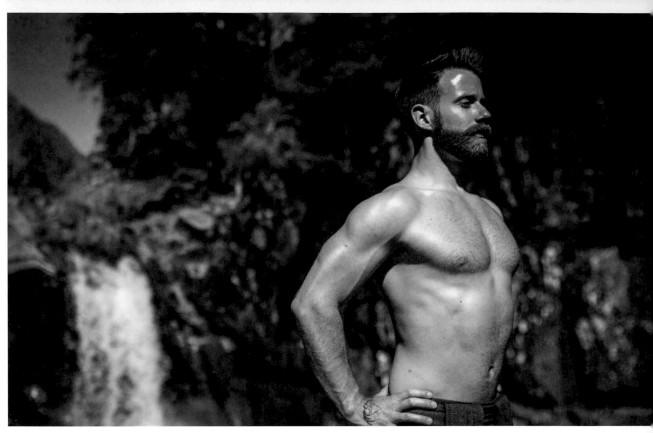

TELESCOPING RIBS

Put your hands on your hips. Inhale to lift the ribs up and away from the pelvis, while tucking your tail bone down.

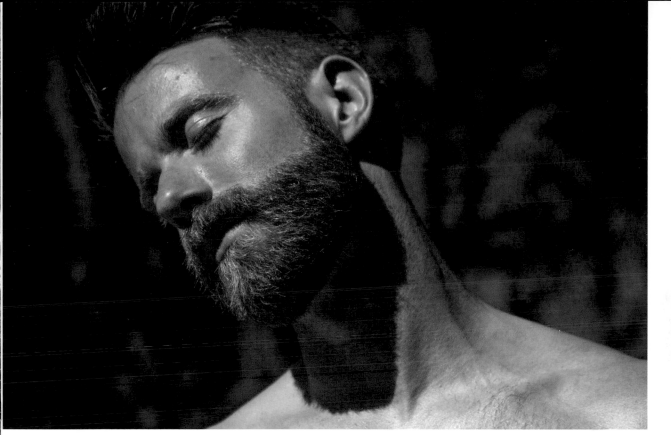

RELAXED NECK | 5 BREATHS PER SIDE

Standing straight, exhale, relaxing your right ear to right
shoulder, feeling where there is tension in the neck. You should
feel a stretch but not pain. Use your right hand to bring your
head back up and repeat on the other side.

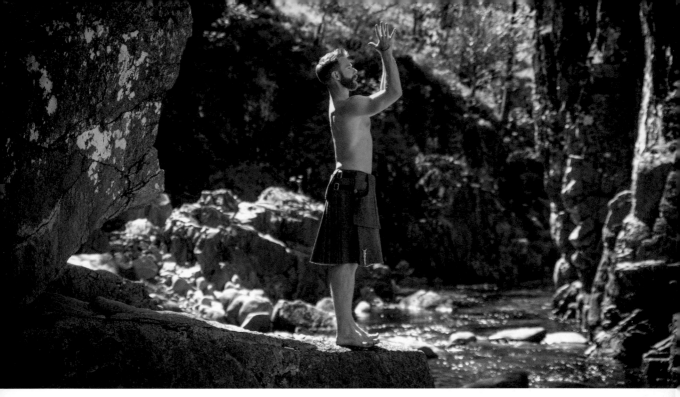

WRAPPED SHOULDERS

Bring both arms up, elbows at shoulder height and forearms parallel. Exhale to reach your elbows forward, sliding your shoulder blades towards your underarms and flexing your chest muscles.

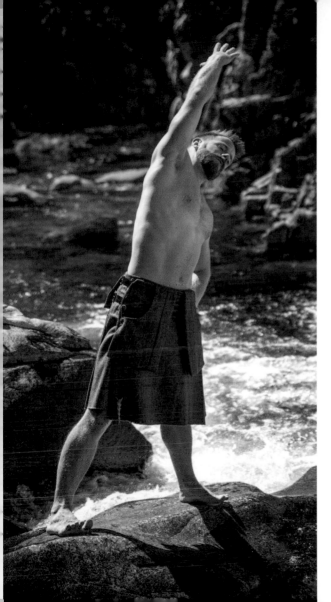

STANDING SIDE BEND | 5 BREATHS PER SIDE

Stand with your feet about 3 feet apart and your left hand
on hip. Inhale, lift the right arm and lean gently to the left
to lengthen the right side of your body. Pull the shoulder blade
towards the underarm as you lean into the side bend. Inhale
to return to centre. Repeat on the other side.

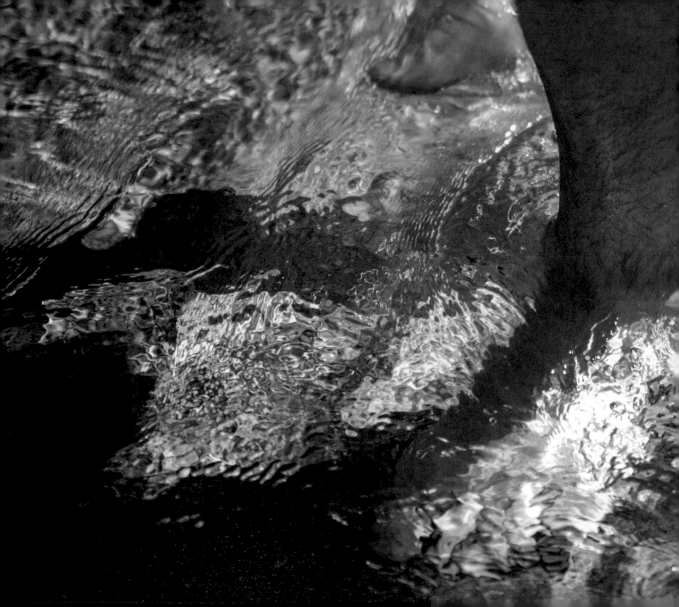

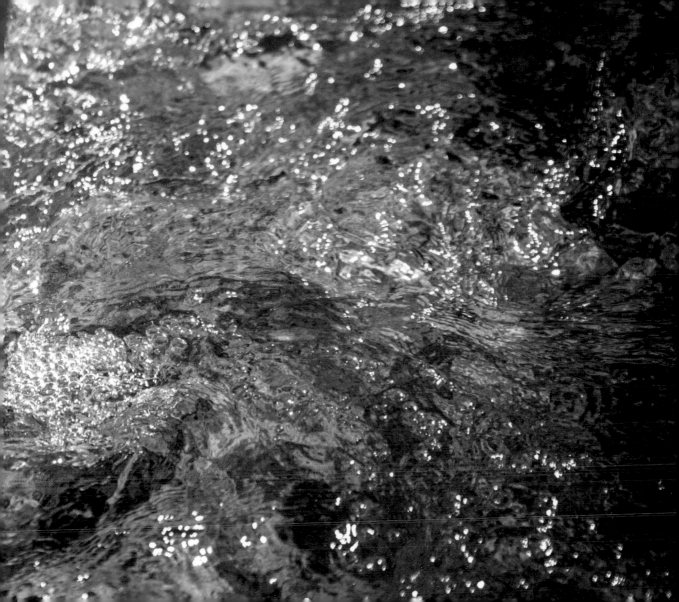

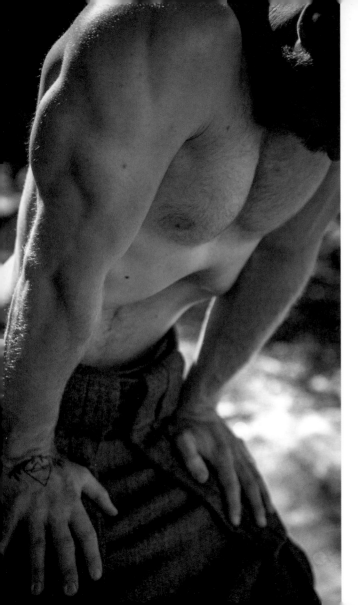

STANDING UDDIYANA | 3 ROUNDS

Stand with your feet hip-distance apart and brace your hands on your upper thighs. Tuck your chin to chest.

Exhale completely through the mouth and, once all the air has been expelled, stretch the ribs away from the pelvis, allowing the belly to pull in. Hold for as long as is comfortable. Relax the belly and inhale.

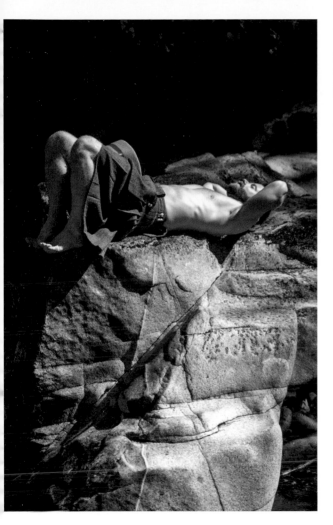

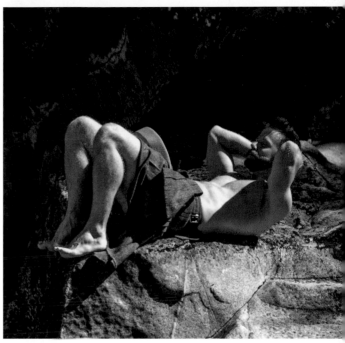

ABS WITH A ROLL | 6 ROUNDS

Place a rolled-up yoga mat or towel between your thighs.
You can do this pose with legs straight up, bent or with your
feet on the ground.

Clasp your hands behind your head. Inhale to press your
lower back down. Hold your breath, tuck the tail bone up and
squeeze the roll. Exhale, lift your head and shoulders up. Inhale,
relax the tail bone and lower the head and shoulders back down.

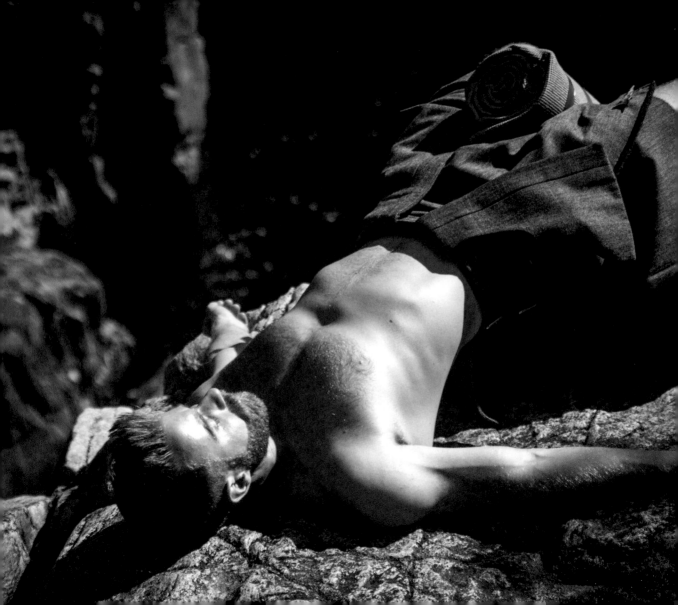

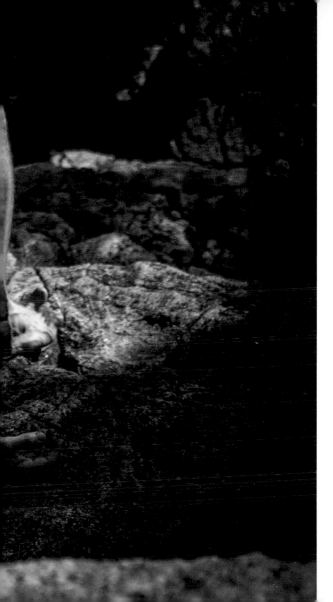

BRIDGE WITH A ROLL | 8–10 BREATHS

Place your feet close to your hips, hip-width apart, and your hands about 1 foot away from your hips, palms facing up. Keeping your neck still, exhale, tuck in your tail bone and lift the pelvis, squeezing the roll. Connect to the strength in your legs. Lower down on an exhale, keeping the tail bone tucked.

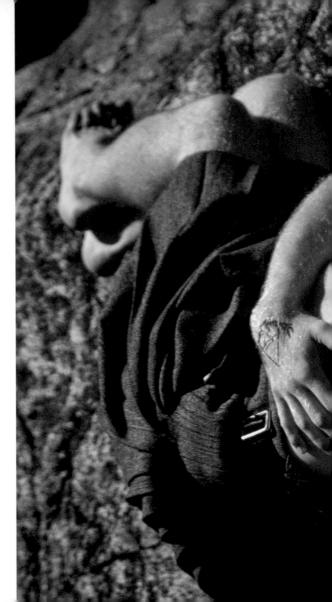

LYING-DOWN SPINAL TWIST | 5 BREATHS PER SIDE

Bring your knees to your chest, arms out in a rugby goalpost
position (elbows bent 90 degrees with forearms parallel).
Exhale and relax your legs over to the right.

Inhale and reach your left arm towards the back of your mat,
right hand on lower ribs. Focus your breath to where your hand is.
Repeat on the other side.

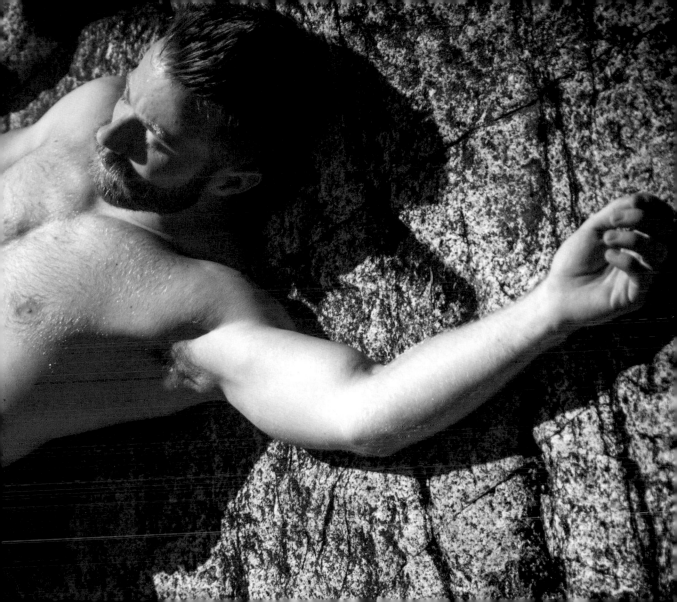

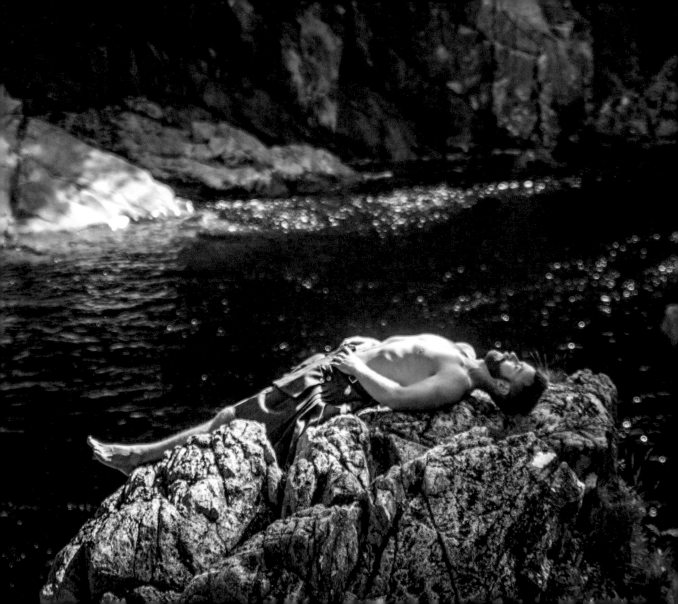

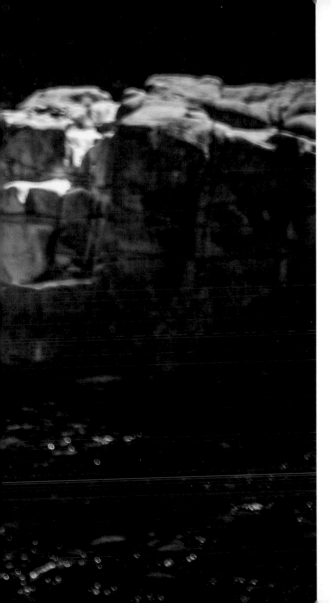

SAVASANA | 4 MINUTES

Resting at the end of a yoga practice is important. In our day-to-day lives, we rarely get time to properly rest, with people trying to get our attention, demanding our time or interrupting our focus. Intentional rest, even for a few minutes, allows you to integrate everything from your yoga practice, to relax and enjoy a set time of intentionally doing nothing. Using a timer can take the anxiety of falling asleep for the afternoon out of your head – been there, done that!

SANCTUARY MEDITATION

Sit or lie somewhere you won't be disturbed. Bring your attention to a place in your mind that you would call your sanctuary; somewhere you feel safe, that gives you a sense of well-being and calm. Imagine a place that supports the feeling of security and ease. Use all of your senses to populate the detail of your sanctuary. Is it a place you have visited? Are there people there? Imagine sounds, sights, sensations and smells that strengthen your connection to this memory or experience. What words would you use to describe what you are sensing? Take your time. Allow your entire body to experience this sanctuary, the feeling of being safe and at ease. Remind yourself that you have the capacity to return to this sanctuary whenever you need to centre yourself and reconnect.

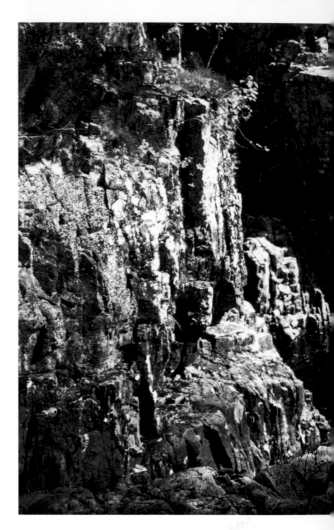

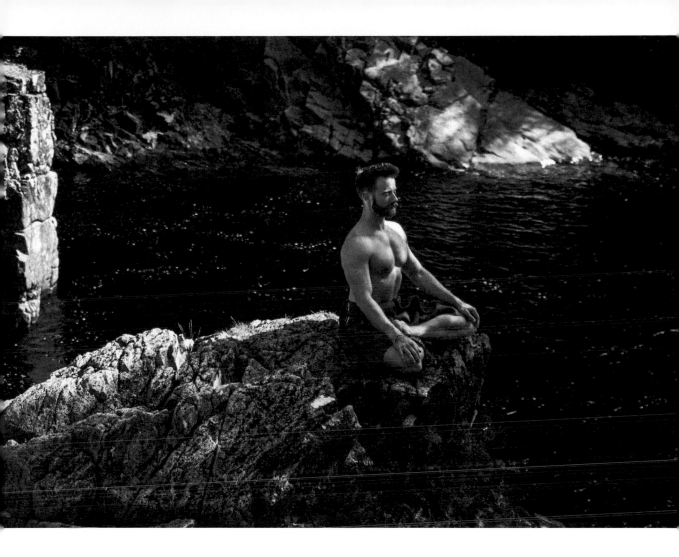

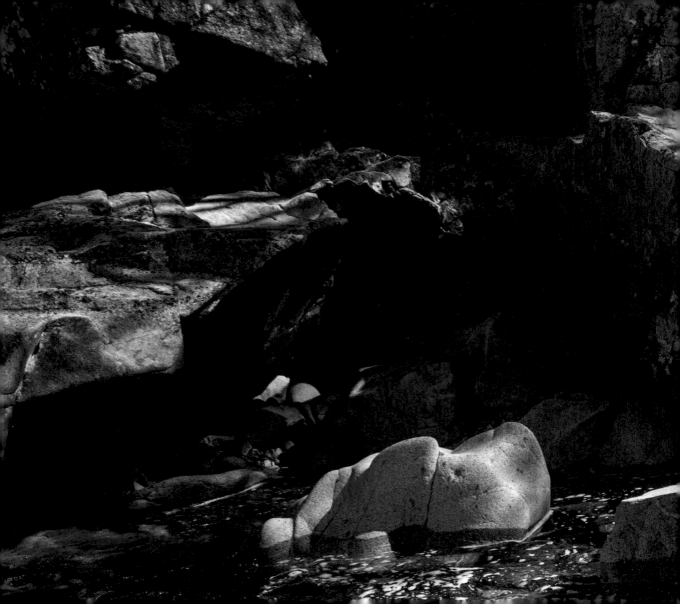

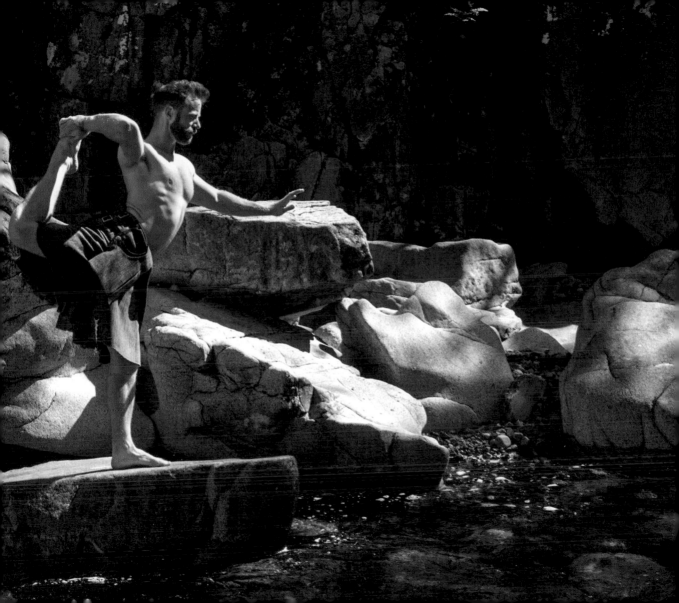

SERENITY

INTENT: TO BE STRUGGLE FREE IN YOUR
BREATH AND MOVEMENT

SERENITY

For a long time in my own yoga practice, I would battle the poses and the struggle became something I wore like a badge of honour. I picked up a lot of injuries and bad habits, and my thinking during my practice was pretty toxic. One day, I was in Lunge pose and I chose not to struggle – it was a revelation. A calm settled over my body, the tension of years ebbed away from my muscles and the pose became a steady place.

In this sequence, use your breath to help you become struggle free. The sequence may be challenging in the beginning, but familiarity is a huge part of being steady. Remind yourself that it's only yoga and you are in no rush. Take a deep breath, feel your feet and let's go.

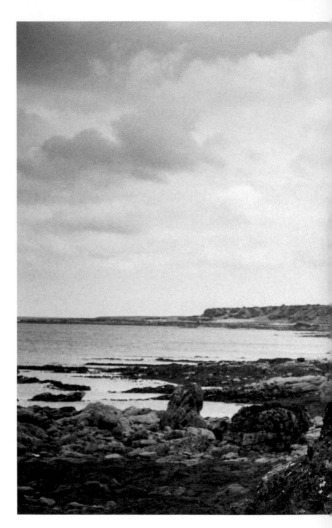

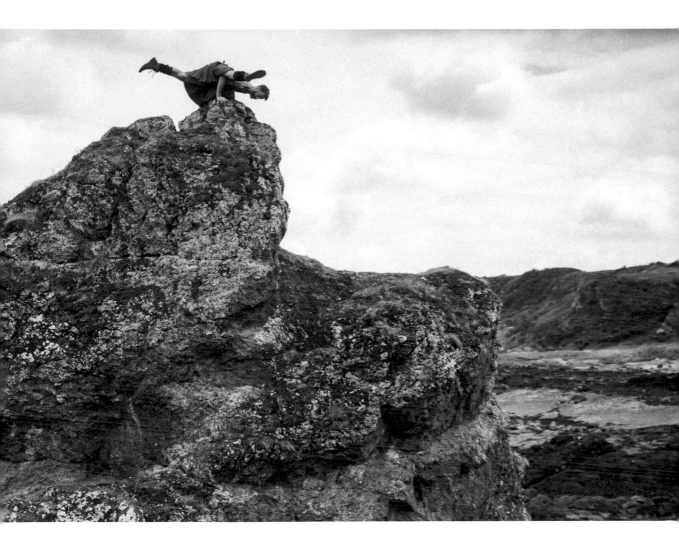

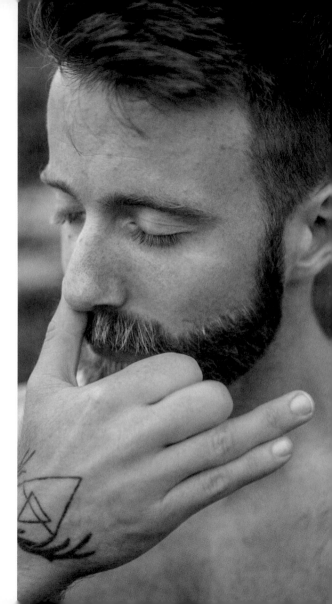

ALTERNATE NOSTRIL BREATHING | 2 ROUNDS

Sitting cross-legged, use your thumb and ring finger of your right hand to open and close the nasal passages.

Closing the right nostril with your thumb, inhale through the left nostril for 10 seconds; hold your breath for 10 seconds, then close the left nostril with your ring finger and exhale through the right nostril for 10 seconds. Inhale through your right nostril for 10 seconds. Hold. Exhale left.

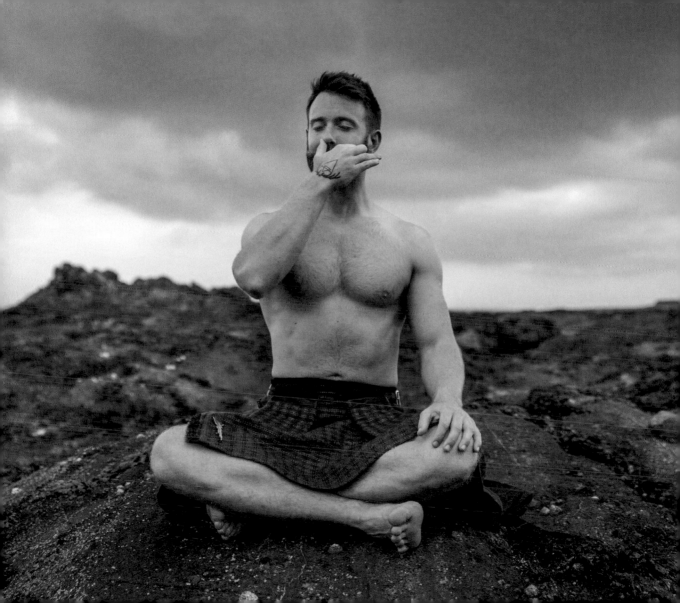

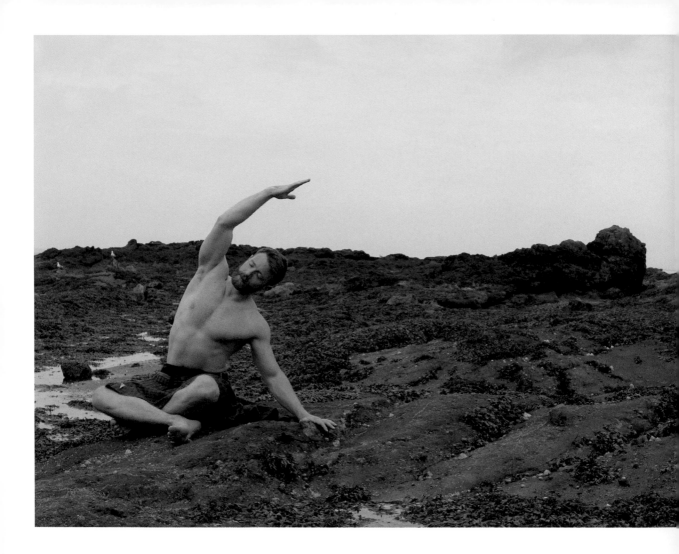

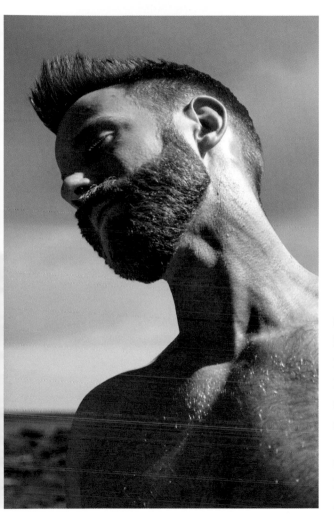

CROSS-LEGGED SIDE BEND WITH NECK RELEASE | 5 BREATHS PER POSITION

Place your left hand on the ground away from your left hip. Inhale and lift the right arm high. Exhale and lean to the left side. Feel the stretch down the right side of your body. Hold for 5 breaths.

Remaining in the pose, move your right arm to the right until about 10 inches from the ground. Exhale to relax your left ear to left shoulder to stretch the neck. Hold for another 5 breaths. Repeat on the other side.

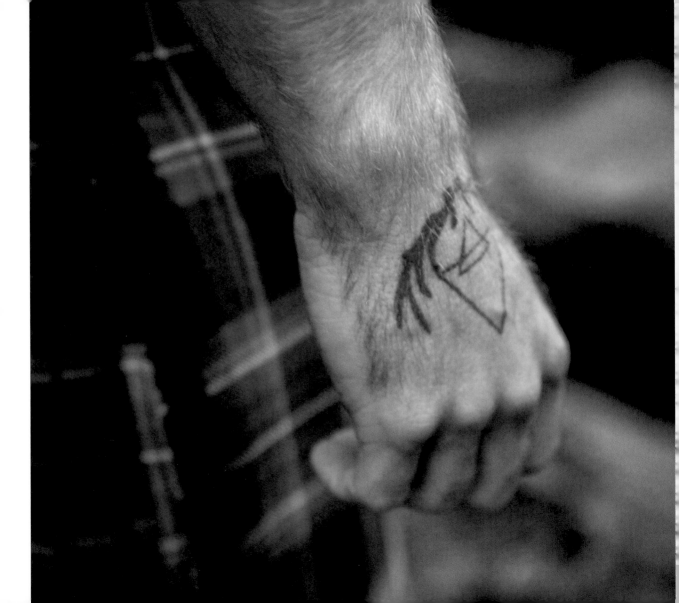

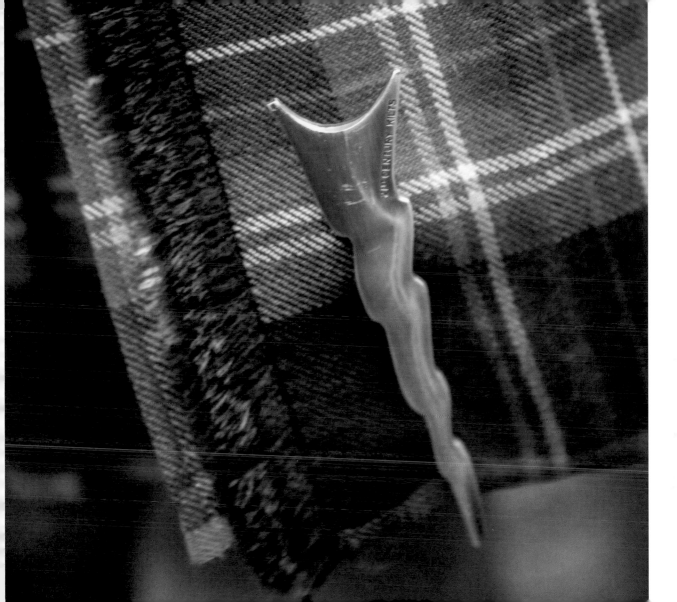

RECLINED HIP SERIES | 5 BREATHS PER POSE

Do all the poses on one side and then repeat on the other side.

KNEE TO CHEST

Lying down, inhale and draw your right knee to your chest. Press the shin against your hands to help spread your back into the ground.

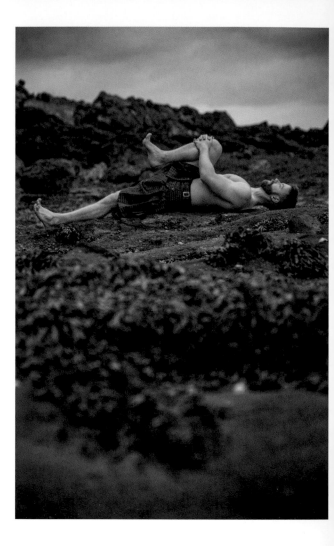

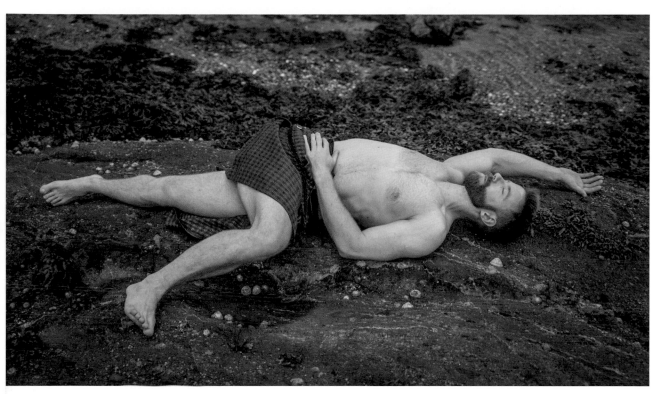

LYING-DOWN TWIST

Begin with the arms in a rugby goalpost position (arms up
with elbows bent 90 degrees and forearms parallel).

Exhale and take the right knee over to the left. Place your
left hand on your lower abdomen. On an inhale come back
to centre.

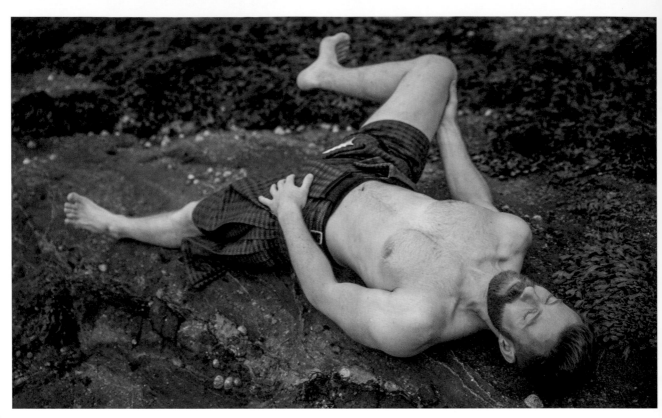

HALF FROG

Stack the right knee above the right hip, with your leg
at a 90-degree angle. Place your left hand on your pelvis
for stability. Exhale and relax the right leg out to the side,
parallel to the ground.

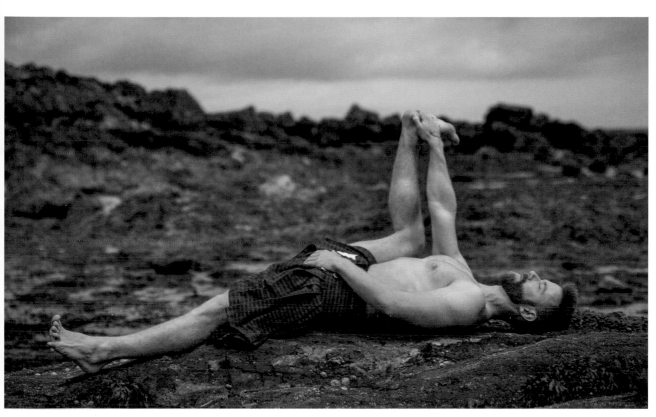

HALF-DEAD BUG

Draw the right knee towards the right underarm, with the leg bent at a 90 degree angle. Hold your ankle or foot with your right hand.

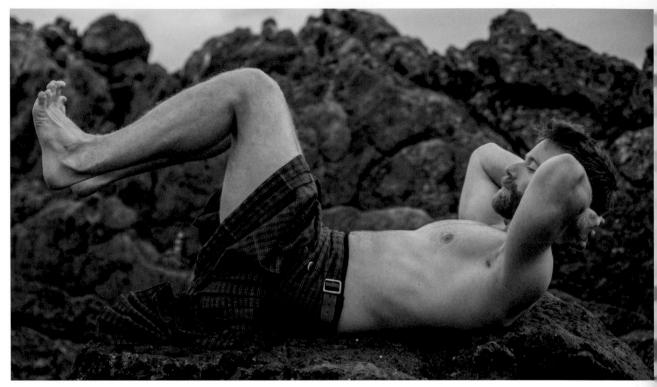

ELBOW TO KNEE | 8 ROUNDS

Lift the knees above the pelvis and clasp your hands behind your
head. Inhale to lift your head and shoulders up. Hold the breath
and tuck the tail bone up. Exhale, straighten your right leg and
reach your elbows towards your left leg, pulling the belly down.
Repeat on the other side. That's one round!

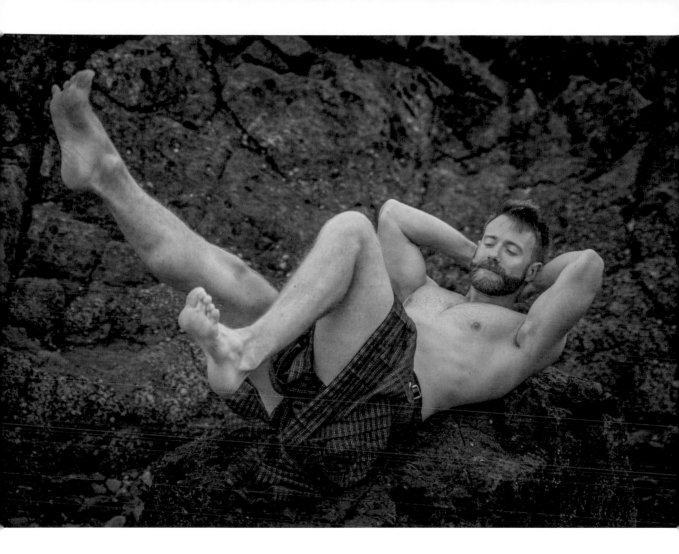

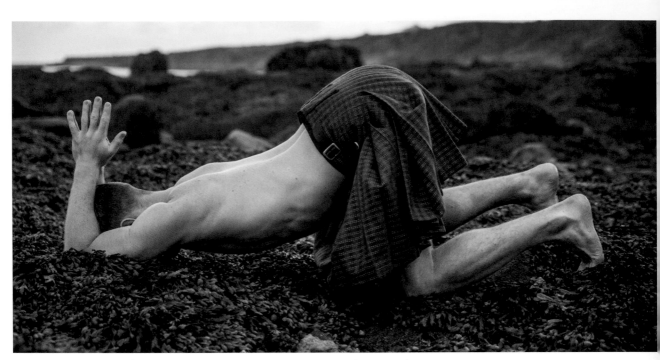

DOLPHIN PRELUDE | 8–10 BREATHS

On your hands and knees, place your elbows 6 inches in front of where your hands were. Hips stay above the knees. Relax your chest towards the ground and bend the elbows.

DOLPHIN | 8–10 BREATHS

Grab your upper arms to ensure that they are shoulder-distance apart. Keeping the elbows where they are, clasp your hands. Inhale to arch the upper back. Exhale to flex your chest muscles and lift your knees – you can keep your knees bent.

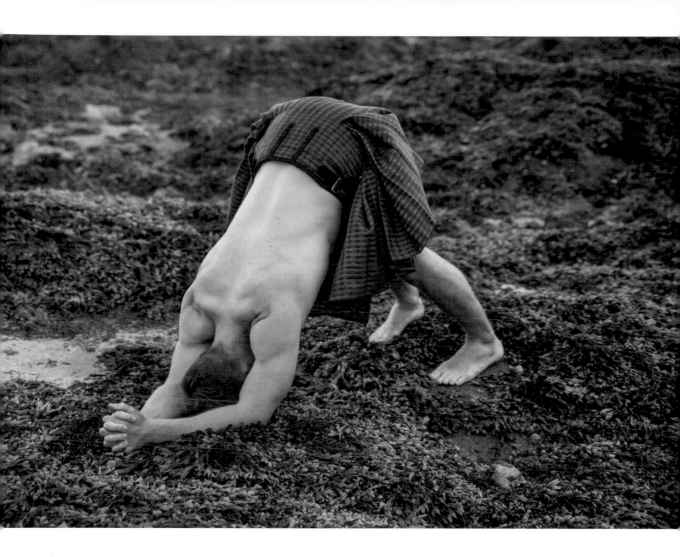

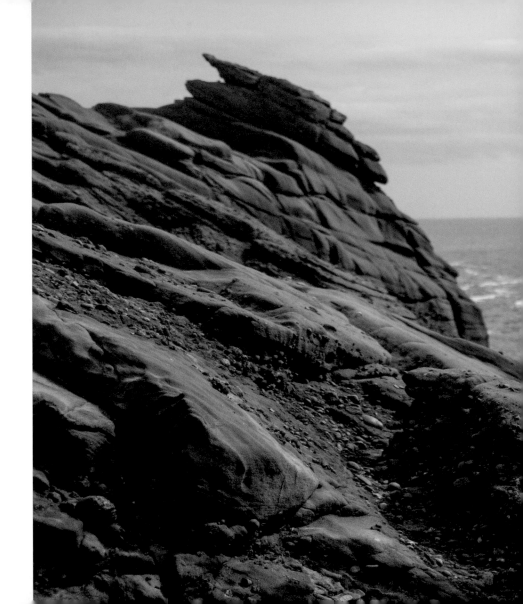

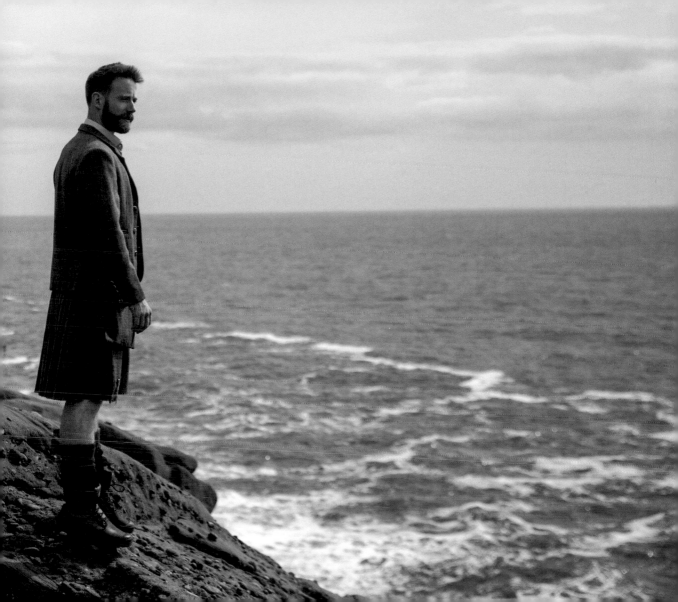

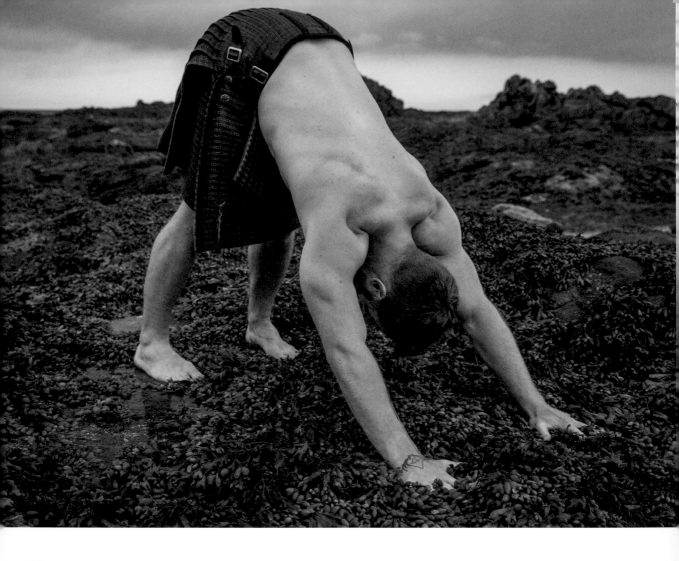

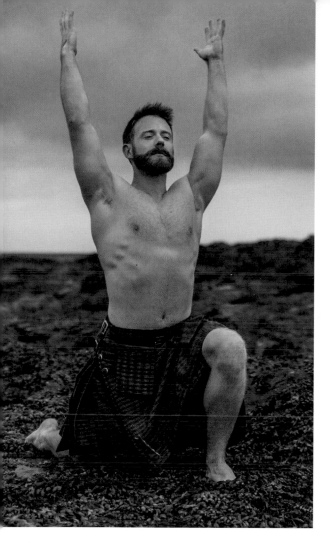

DOWNWARD-FACING DOG TO LUNGE

From all fours, tuck your toes under and lift your hips, taking them back into Downward-facing Dog. (Your body should be the shape of an upside-down 'V'). Wrap the shoulder blades towards the underarms.

Exhale, step the left foot forwards between your hands and lower the hips into Lunge. Keep the front foot flat, bend your left knee deeply and keep the right knee down.

Inhale, lift your arms up and tuck the tail bone down. After 5 breaths, set hands down and go back to Downward-facing Dog. Repeat, stepping your right foot forwards into Lunge.

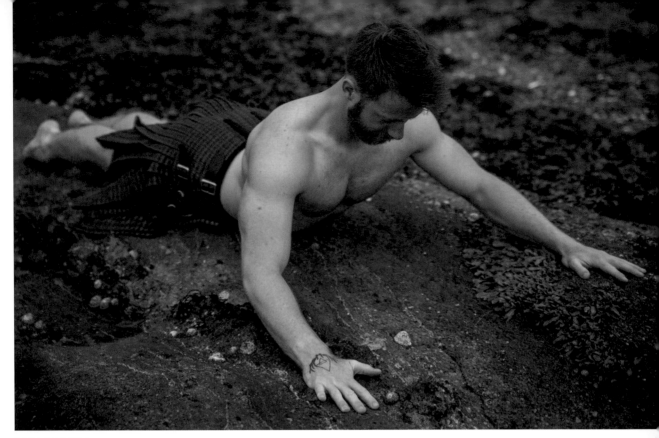

LOW COBRA | 5 BREATHS

Legs together, move your elbows a little in front of your
shoulders. Inhale to lift the chest. Pull the chest forwards and
arms backwards so the elbows lift. Exhale to tuck the tail bone
and press down through the feet, engaging your legs.

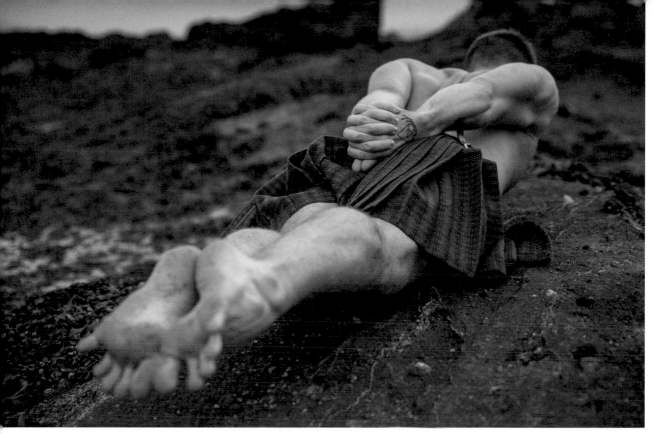

BOAT | 5 BREATHS

Clasp your hands at your lower back. Inhale to lift the chest and
legs. Exhale, draw shoulder blades towards each other and tuck
your tail bone.

BADDHA KONASANA ON THE BACK | 8–10 BREATHS

Bring the feet either above the chest or on the ground.

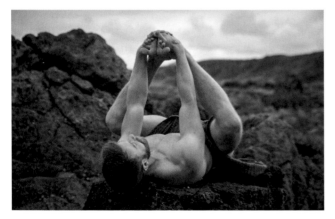

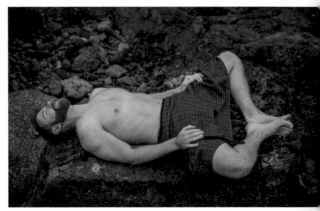

FEET UP

Press lower back down and hold your feet.

FEET DOWN

Gently push hands against your legs to keep the spine long.

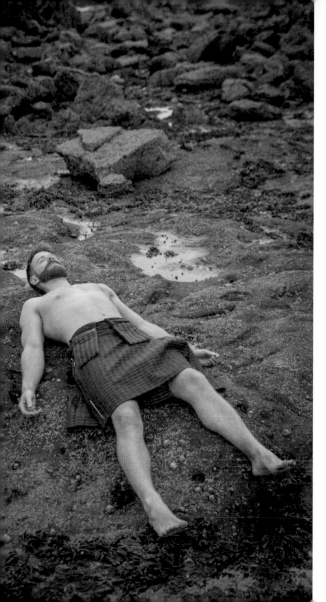

SAVASANA

Palms facing up. Legs flopped out to the sides. Relax completely.

SENSORY MEDITATION

You can do this in your office or at home but outside in nature this takes on a life of its own as you begin to feel a connection to the web of life. Sitting comfortably, with your eyes open or closed, open your senses to the environment around you.

Listen to the sounds you can hear in the distance. Listen to the sounds nearer to you. Sense the air on your skin. Sense where your body is in contact with the ground. Sense the textures of what is supporting you. Sense if there is the presence of cold or warmth. Sense the colours you can see, the objects around you, the objects closer to you. Sense the feel of your clothes on your skin. Observe how your body and mind have reacted to welcoming the environment around you. What else can you sense in this open state?

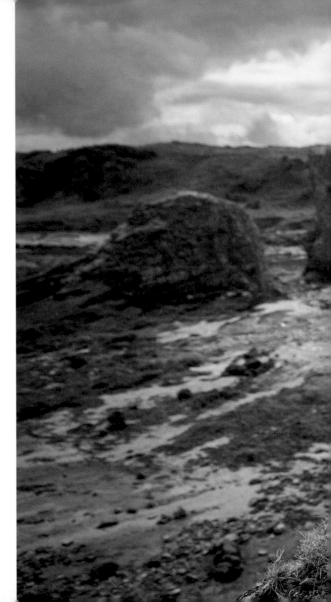

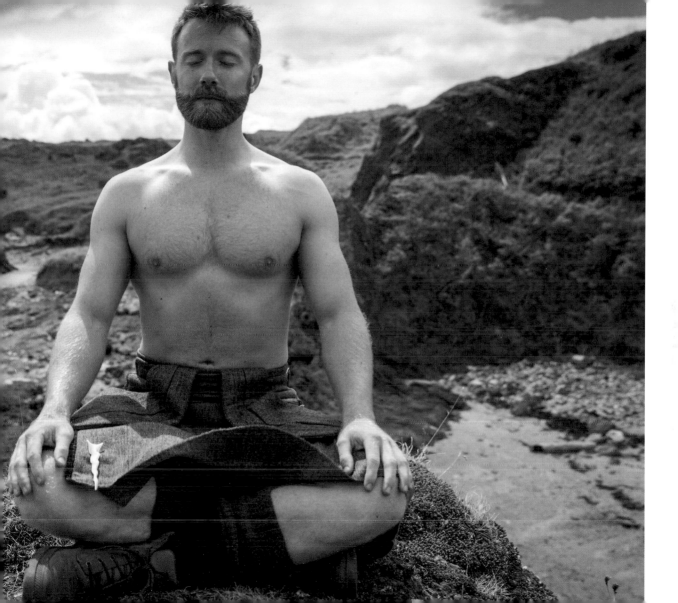

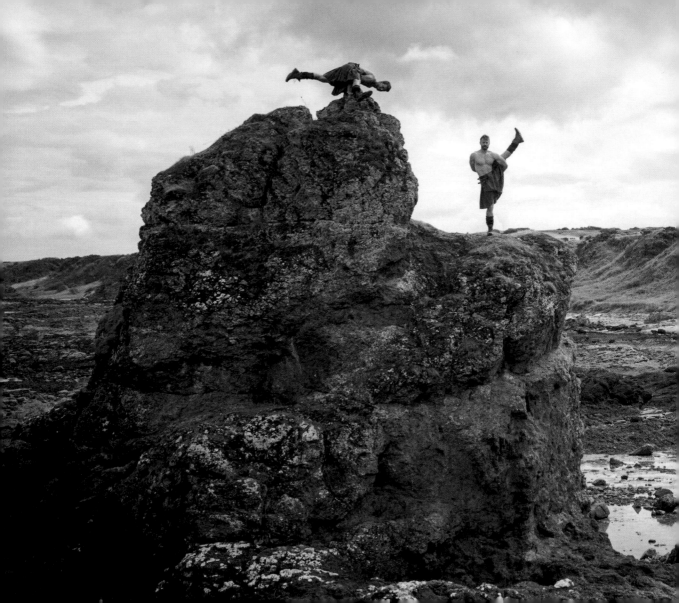

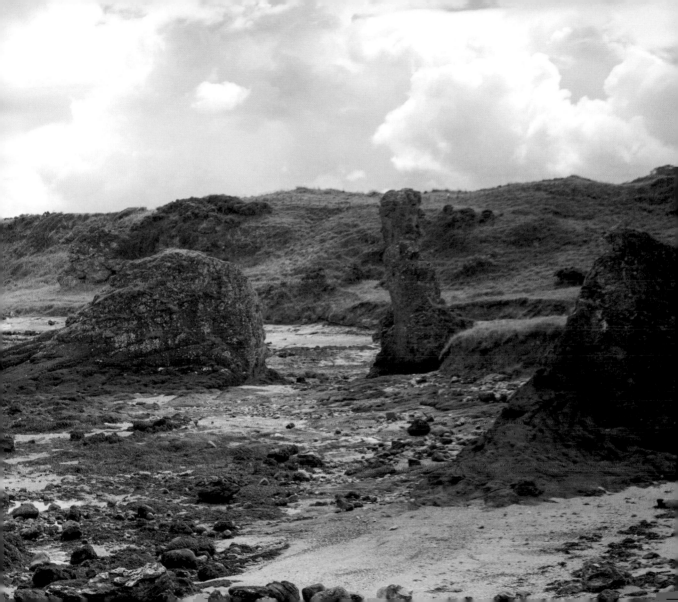

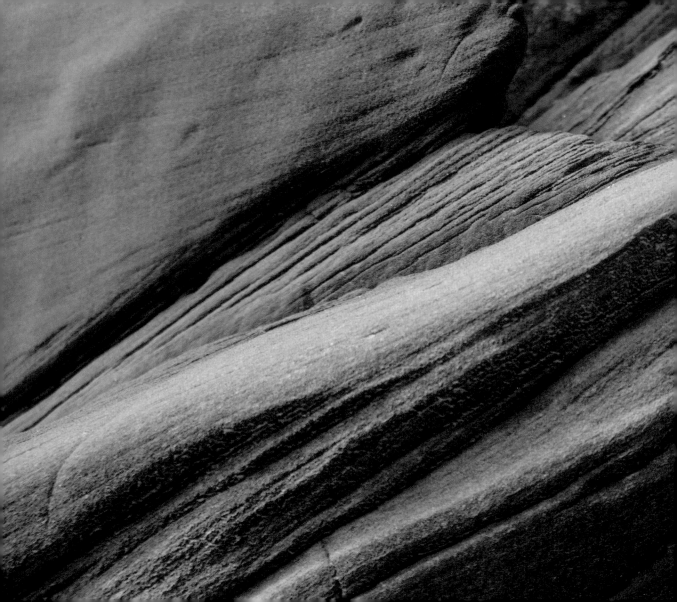

STRENGTH

INTENT: TO CONNECT TO THE STRENGTH IN YOUR LEGS

STRENGTH

This sequence builds on the foundations we have been creating to help you feel the strength and support that you can create for yourself. After the Sun Salutations we move into a standing pose series which gets you holding the poses all on one side before changing. Standing poses invite you to get steady on your legs and sense your quitting points. But instead of quitting, what if you did something different? Maybe modify the pose, or do a few exhales through your mouth. Begin to turn the fire of the poses into an ally!

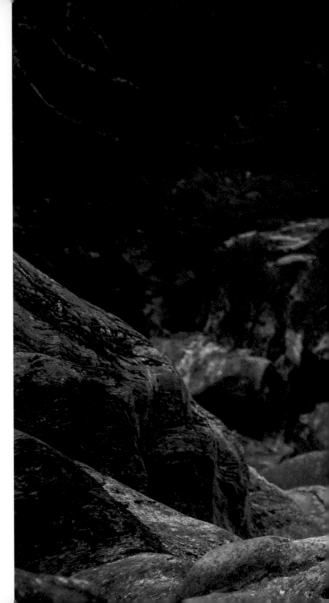

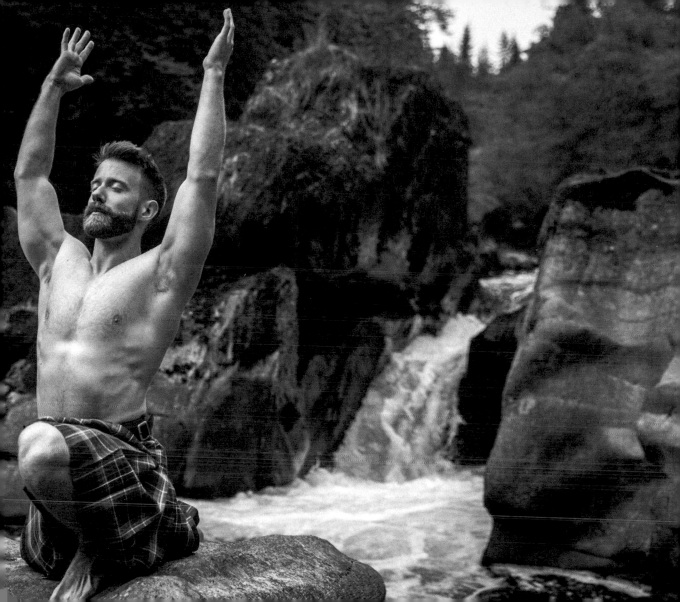

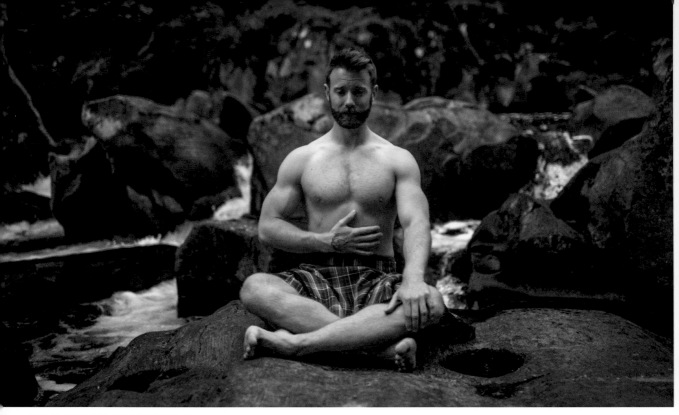

KAPALABHATI BREATHING | 50 ROUNDS

As if gently blowing your nose, sharply contract naval to spine
to exhale a short blast of air, and quickly release to let the inhale
come in.

Repeat with one hand on your abdomen to feel the
contraction. Keep the pace steady and rhythmic without force.

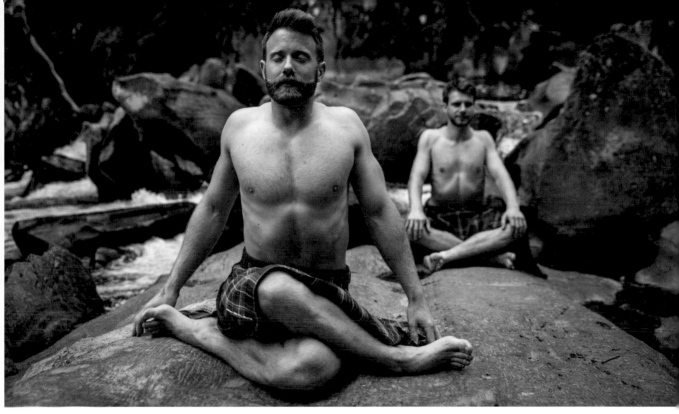

KNEE PILE SHOULDER SHRUGS | 2 ROUNDS

Cross right leg over left, feet pointing back. (Straighten the
top leg if difficult.) Inhale and bring shoulders up by your ears.
Exhale, squeeze the shoulders back and drag down. Repeat two
more times.

    Change the cross of your legs for the second round.

OPTION: *Sit cross-legged.*

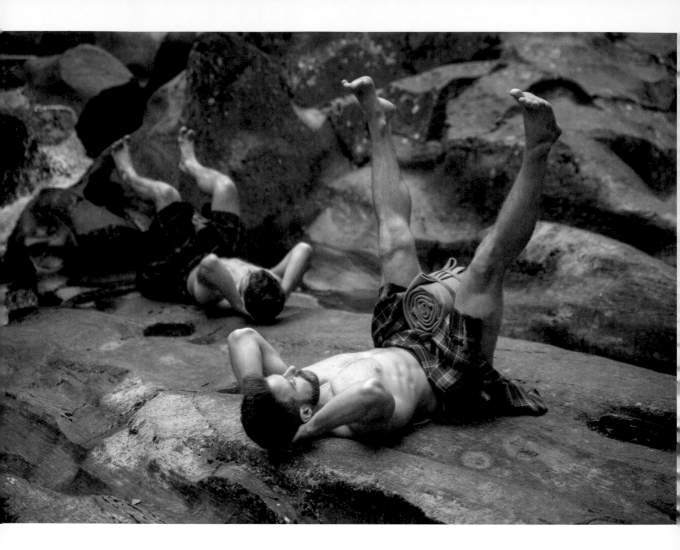

ABS WITH A ROLL | 8 ROUNDS

Place a rolled-up yoga mat or towel between your thighs.
Do this either with your legs straight up, bent or with your
feet on the ground. Clasp your hands behind your head.

Inhale to press your lower back down. Hold your breath,
tuck your tail bone up and squeeze the roll. Exhale, lift head
and shoulders up. Inhale, relax the tail bone and lower the
head and shoulders back down.

OPTION: *Legs bent will take the pressure off the legs and lower back.*
For lower back injuries, brace the feet against a wall.

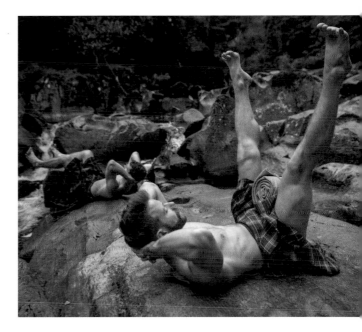

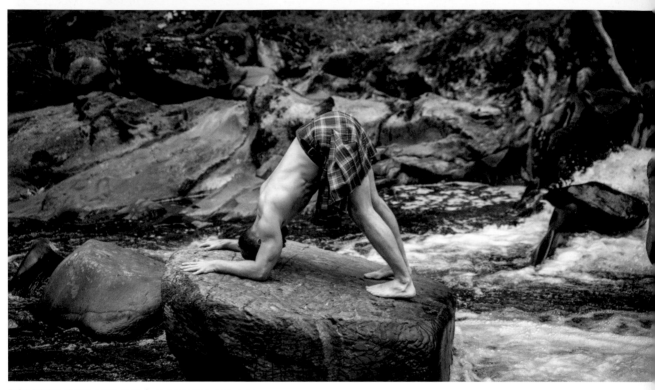

DOLPHIN ONE LEG UP | 5 BREATHS PER LEG

Grab your upper arms to ensure that they are shoulder-distance apart. Place the hands forward. Inhale to arch the upper back. Exhale to flex your chest muscles and lift knees – you can keep knees bent. Inhale to lift your right leg up without collapsing in the lower back. Repeat with the left leg.

OPTION: *Clasp your hands if you have a shoulder or neck injury.*

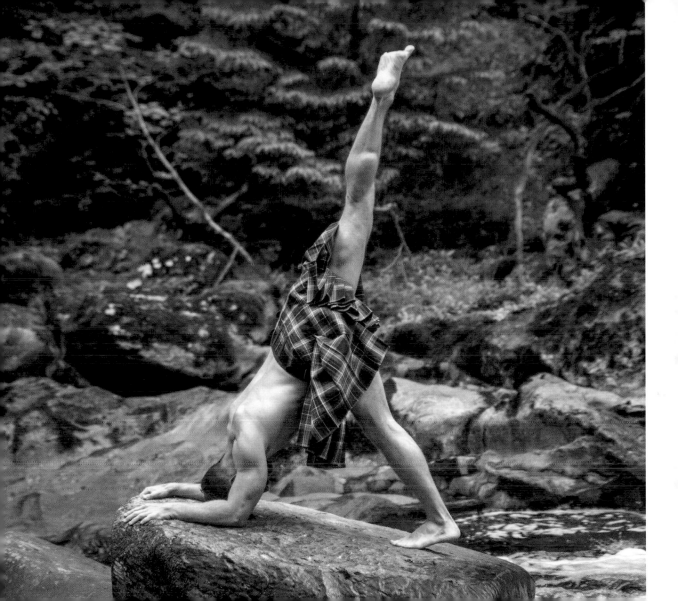

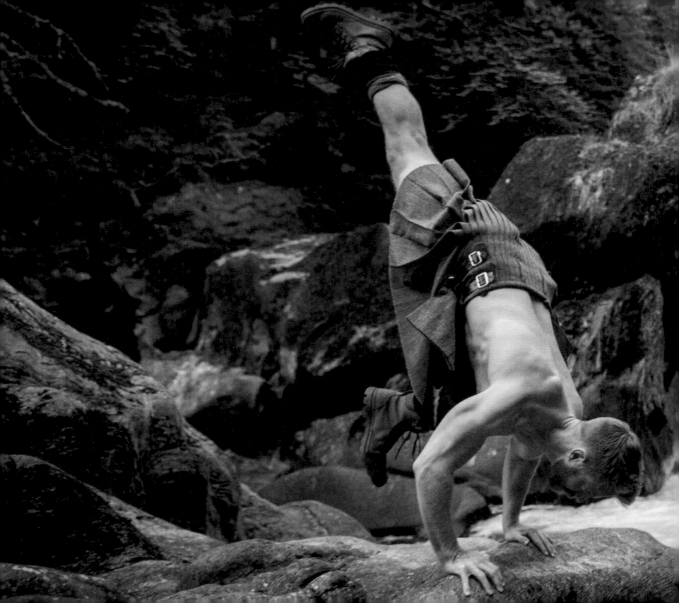

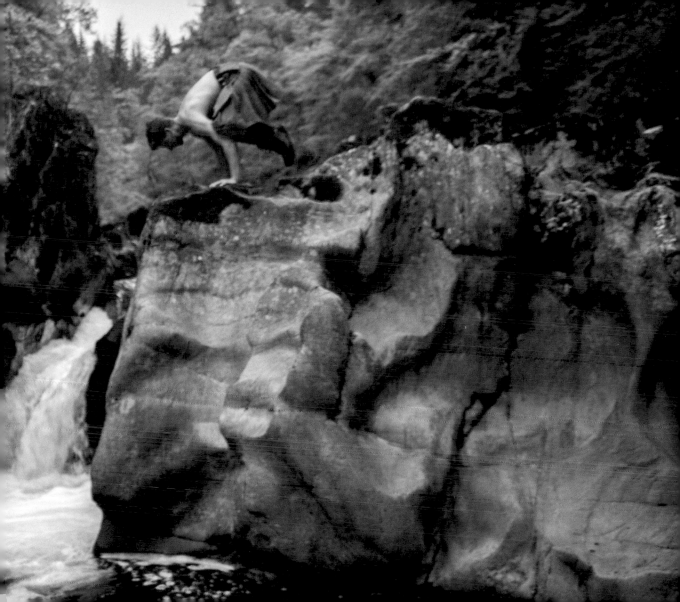

SUN SALUTATION | 4 ROUNDS

Standing, Arms Up, Forward Bend, Lunge, Plank, Low
Cobra, Downward-facing Dog, Lunge, Forward Bend,
Arms Up, Standing.

Inhale, Arms Up.

Exhale, Forward Bend.

Inhale, step left foot back into Lunge.

Exhale, take right foot back into Plank. Lower to ground.

Inhale, Low Cobra.

Exhale, Downward-facing Dog.

Inhale, step left foot forward into Lunge.

Exhale, bring right foot to meet left. Forward Bend.

Inhale, Arms Up.

Exhale, hands to chest.

(Alternate the legs in Lunge pose for each round.)

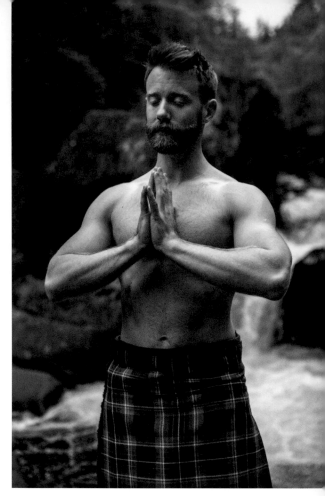

STANDING

Tuck the tail bone down and feel your active feet.

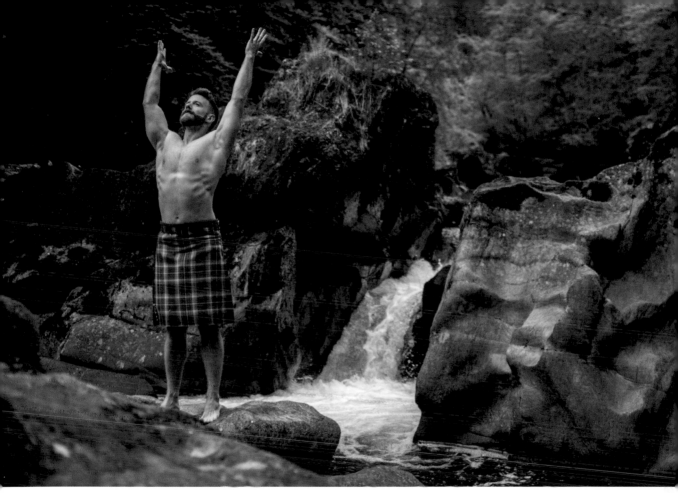

ARMS UP

Inhale to reach arms up while engaging through your thighs.

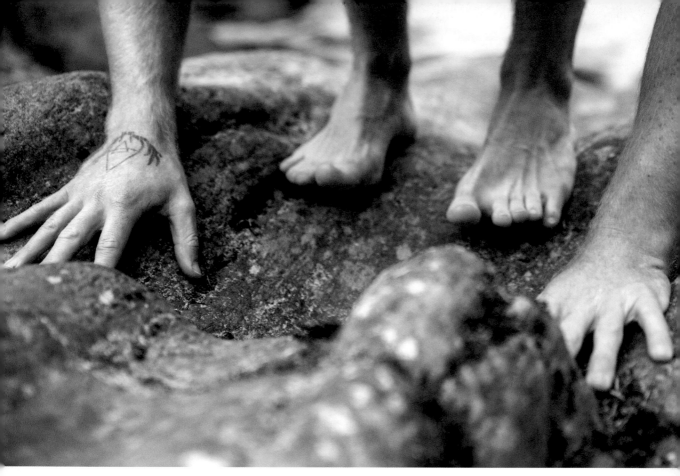

FORWARD BEND

Exhale to bend forward with knees bent and neck relaxed.

As you get more flexible, work with straighter legs.

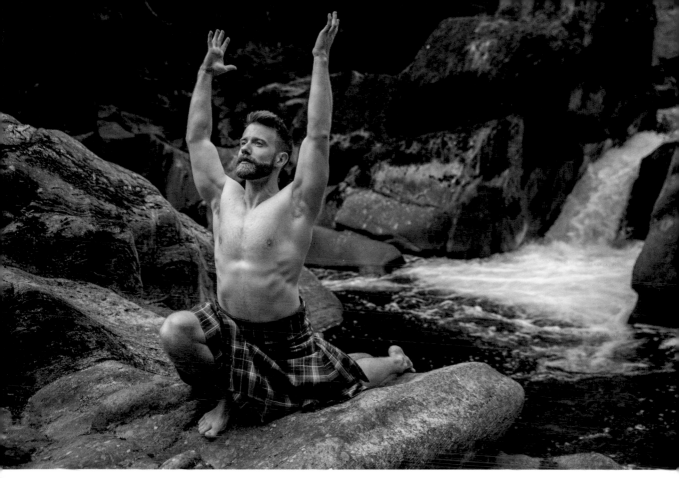

LUNGE

Inhale to Lunge pose, arms up. Keep the feet active.

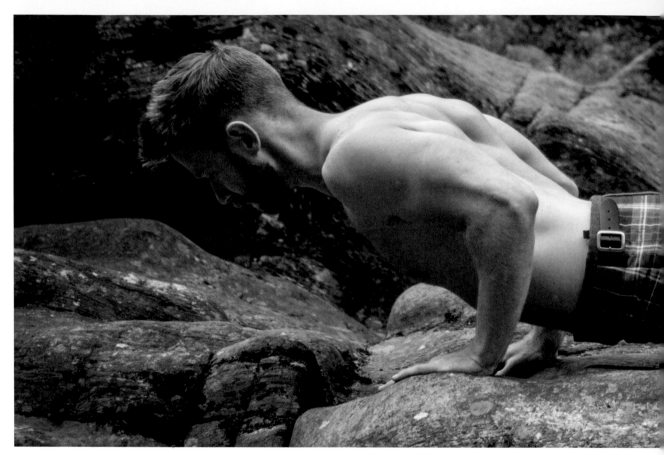

PLANK

Exhale to Plank pose. Lower your torso to the ground with
your knees down.

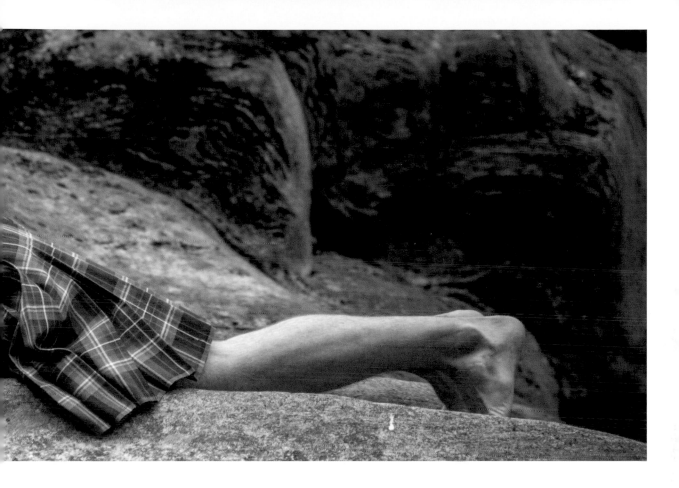

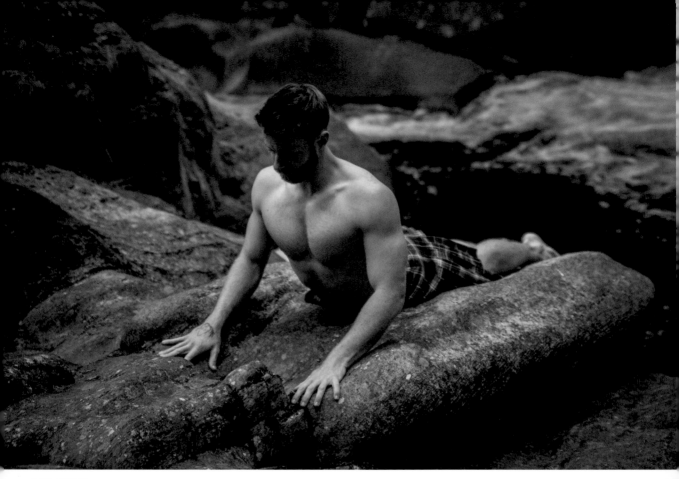

LOW COBRA

Inhale to Low Cobra pose. Pull the chest forwards and tuck the
tail bone towards your heels.

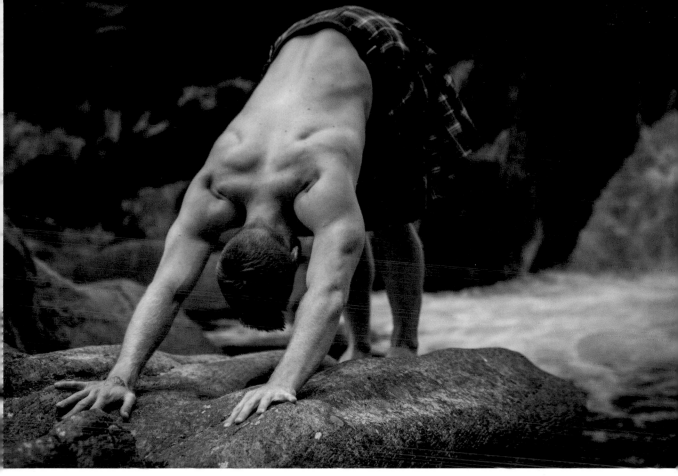

DOWNWARD—FACING DOG

Exhale to Downward-facing Dog pose. Lift the knees up and
wrap your shoulder blades towards the underarms.

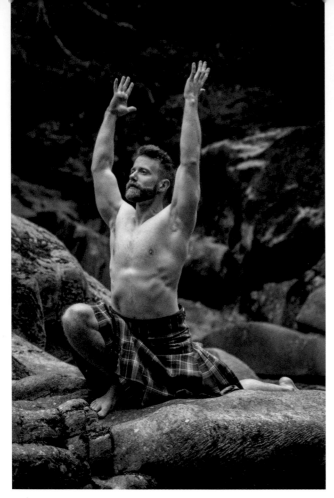

LUNGE

Inhale to Lunge pose, arms up.

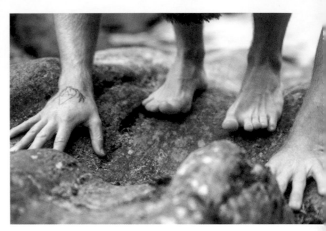

FORWARD BEND

Exhale to bend forward, knees bent.

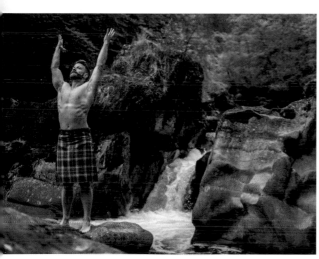

ARMS UP

Inhale to reach up.

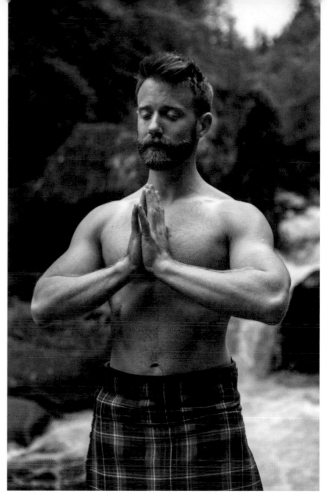

STANDING

Exhale to bring your hands together at your chest.

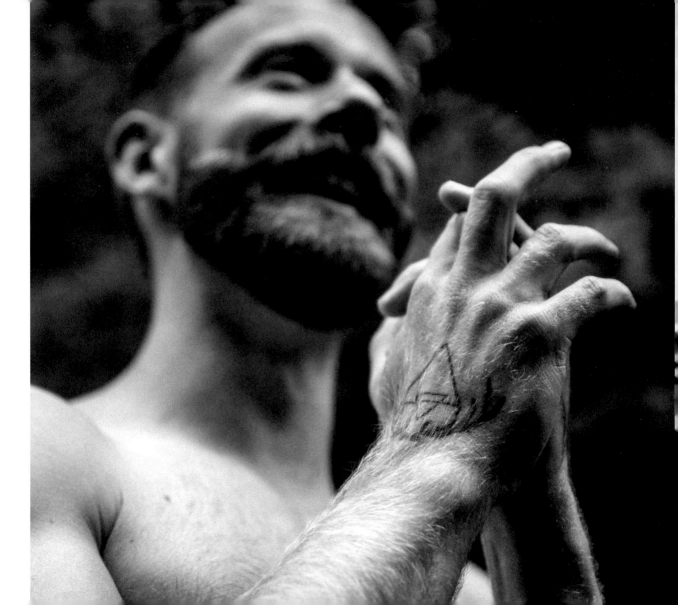

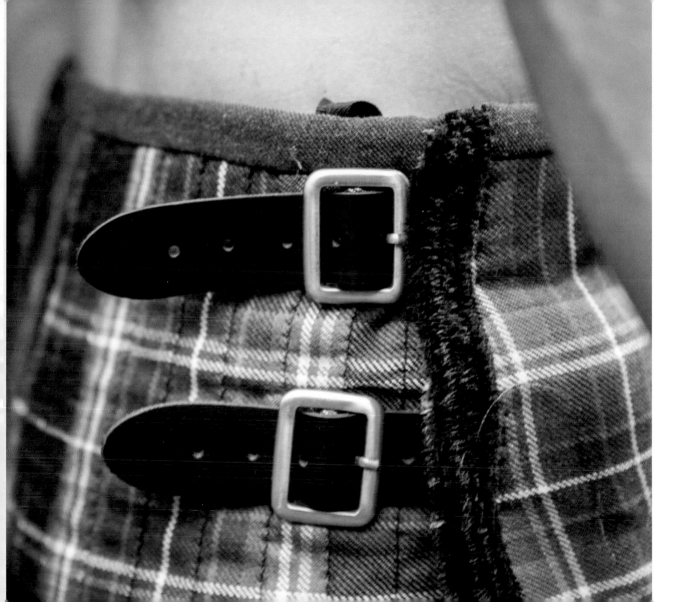

STANDING SEQUENCE | 5 BREATHS PER POSE

Do all the poses on one side and then repeat on the other side.

WARRIOR II

Feet about 4 feet apart and parallel. Turn the left foot
forwards. Exhale to bend the left leg to 90 degrees.
Inhale, lift the arms up parallel to the ground.

OPTION: *Press your hands into your hips to elongate the spine.*

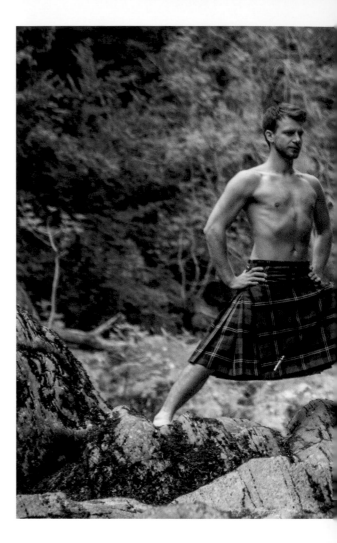

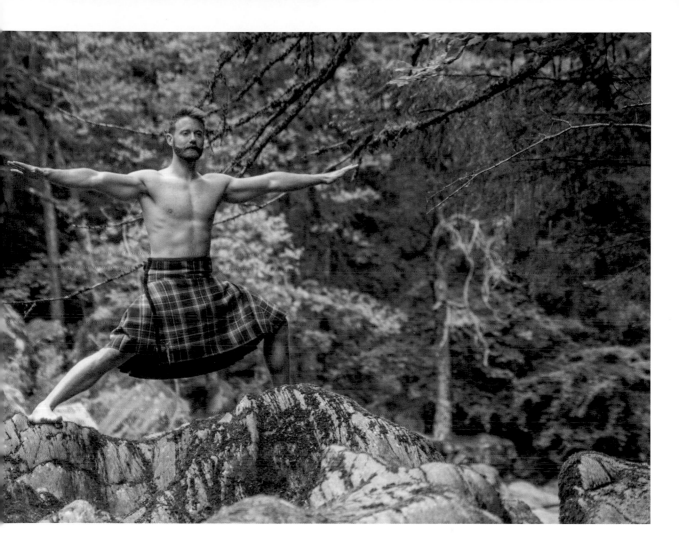

REVERSE WARRIOR

From Warrior II, inhale to place your right arm on the right leg. Exhale to lean over the right leg and reach the left arm overhead.

OPTION: *Reach the left arm towards the left knee and relax your neck.*

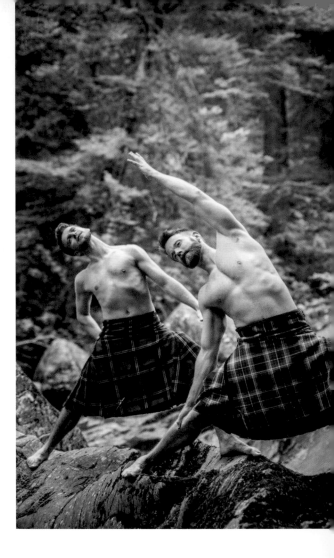

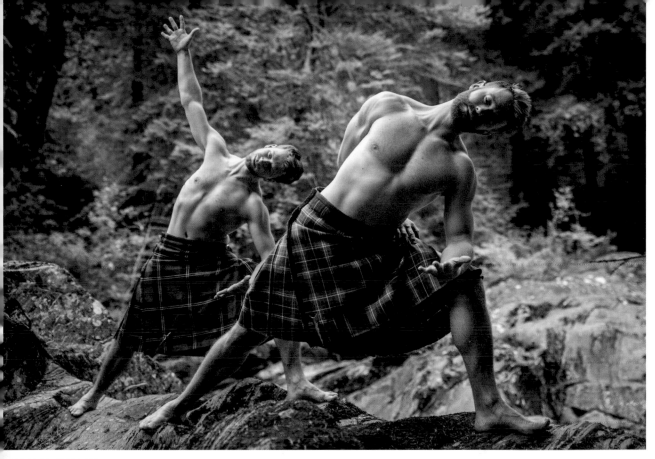

EXTENDED WARRIOR

Return to Warrior II. Exhale to set your left forearm onto the left leg, right arm behind the back to hold inner left thigh or waistband. Relax your neck.

OPTION: *Reach the arm up with active hands to work with a stiff shoulder.*

EASY TWISTING WARRIOR

Set the right hand down under the shoulder to the right of the left foot. The right heel is up. Inhale to twist the left arm up. Lift through the right leg and extend through the arms.

OPTION: *Set the right knee down.*

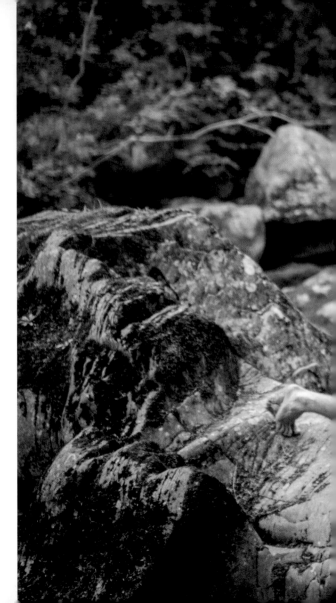

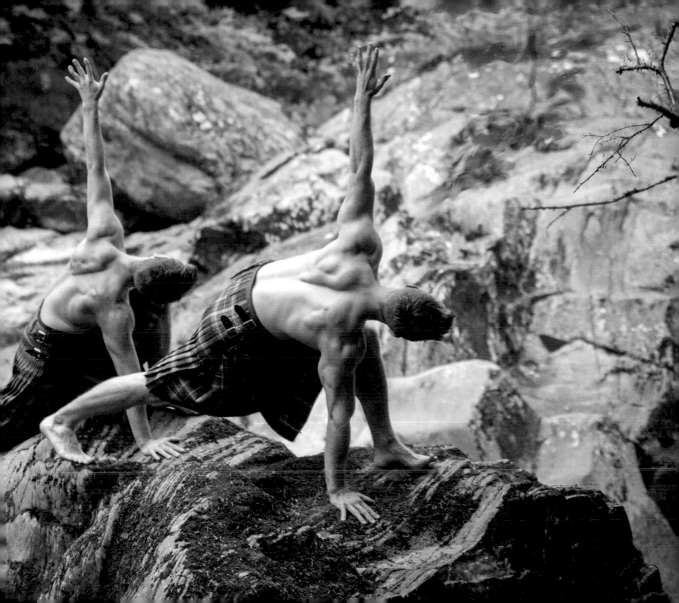

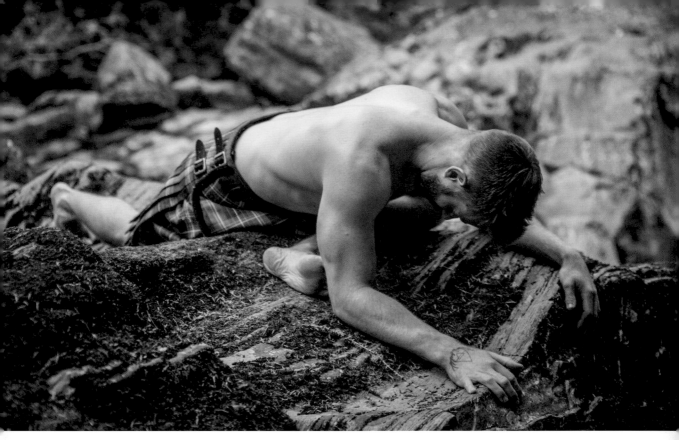

PIGEON

Place the left foot towards the right hip and lower down to
elbows or arms. Relax. As your hips open, if there is no pressure
on the knee, you can move the left foot closer to your elbow,
bringing the shin parallel to the front of the mat.

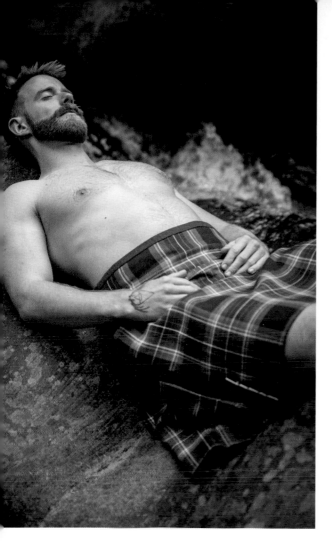

SAVASANA

Another way to meditate is with your legs raised against a wall. Place your hips a few inches from the wall and rest with the legs either straight up or in straddle.

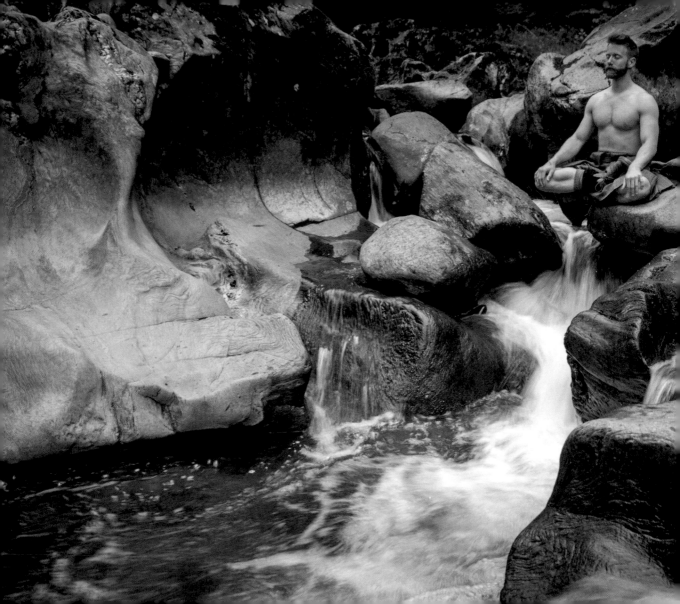

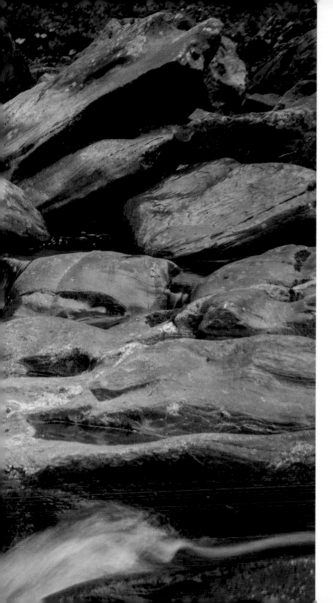

BREATHING MEDITATION

With this exercise, if you lose focus or get distracted, start again from the count of one and use it to increase your resilience for staying attentive. Initially, do this in a quiet place where you won't be disturbed.

Count your breaths as follows: Inhale, ribcage expanding: one. Exhale, belly pulls in: one. Inhale, ribcage expanding: two … Repeat this up to the count of ten and then begin again. If you reach ten, take a moment to feel the effect this has had on your body and mind. You will, with practice, be able to do this breath count anywhere!

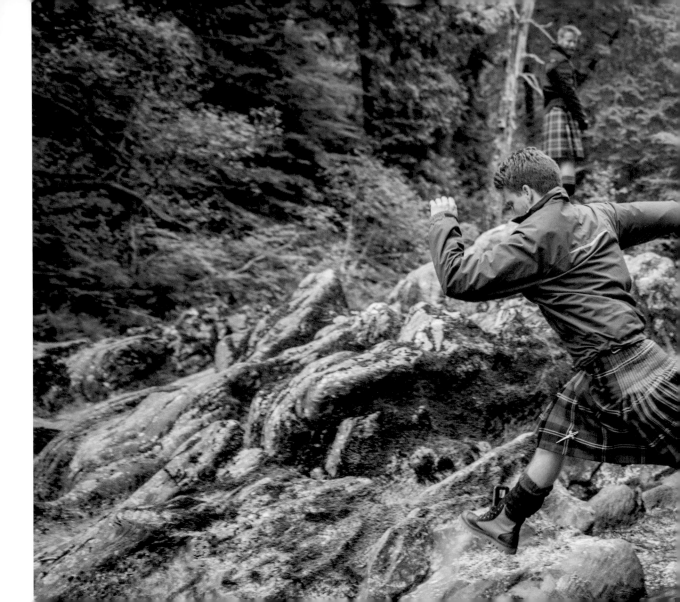

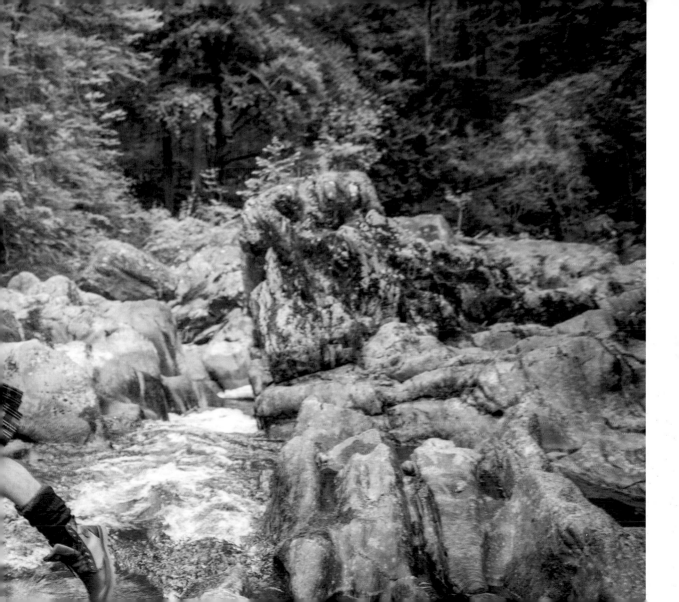

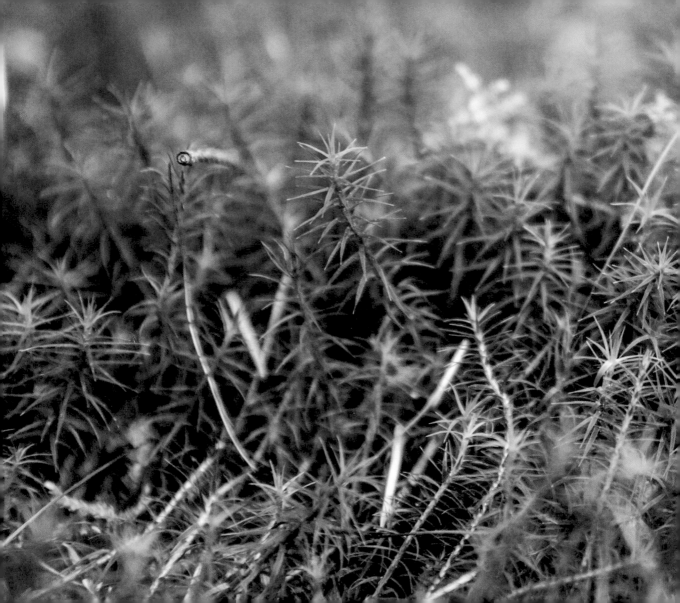

POWER

INTENT: TO EXPLORE THE FIRST EDGE OF YOUR RESISTANCE
AND WAIT FOR IT TO SHIFT BEFORE GOING DEEPER

POWER

An advanced practice isn't about achieving big poses or holding them for ages; it is about giving yourself what you need in each moment, in each pose and in each breath. The fourth sequence gives you an opportunity to connect to your power while also feeling for the moments of letting go. When you come up against resistance in the poses, get steady on your feet and breathe deeply until the first edge of resistance shifts. By being patient in these moments you hold space for new pathways to open up.

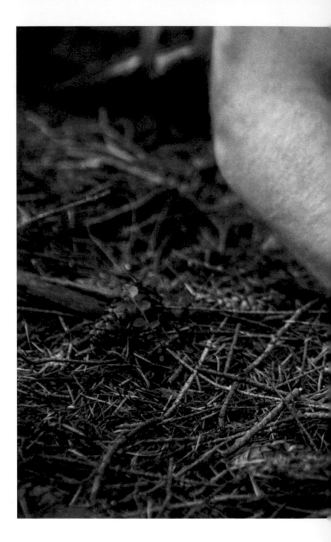

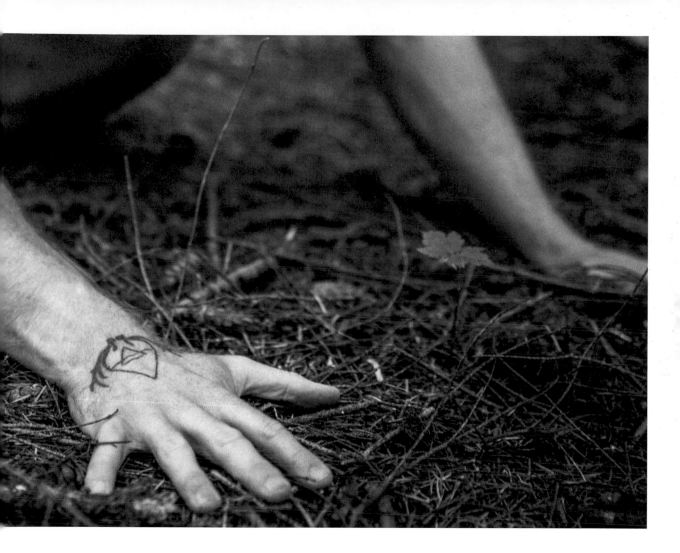

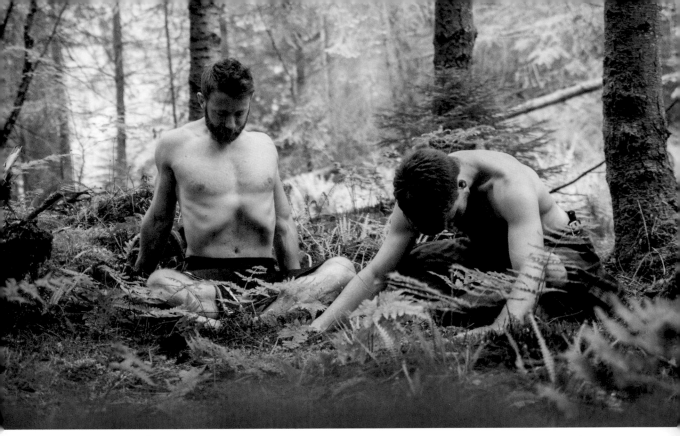

SEATED UDDIYANA | 3 ROUNDS

Brace your arms on the ground. Inhale deeply and hold your breath. Exhale everything out and hold your breath. Scoop ribs up and flare ribs. Hold for a count of ten. Release the belly and inhale.

OPTION: *If comfortable for the lower back, fold forwards over the legs on the exhale.*

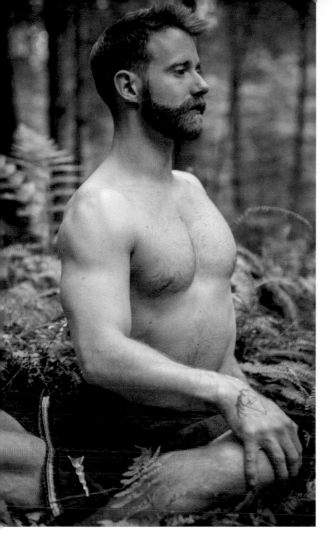

CROSS-LEGGED SPINAL TWIST | 5 BREATHS PER SIDE

Set your right hand to left knee and left hand behind the back. Inhale to telescope your ribs up. Exhale to twist the torso to the left, chin in line with chest. On an exhale return to centre. Repeat on the other side.

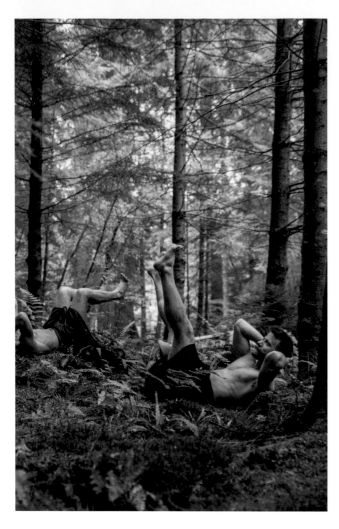

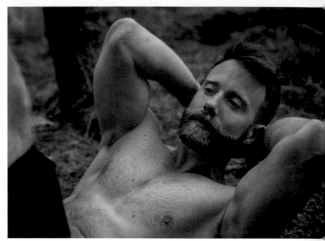

TWISTING ABS WITH A ROLL | 4 ROUNDS

Place the roll between your inner thighs. Clasp your hands behind your head. Lift head and shoulders up. Inhale into the lower back. Hold your breath, squeeze the roll. Exhale, tuck the tail bone, reach elbows to left knee. Inhale back to centre. Repeat towards the right knee to complete one round.

OPTION: *Work with the legs bent to take the pressure off the lower back. Or, for lower back injuries, brace the feet against a wall.*

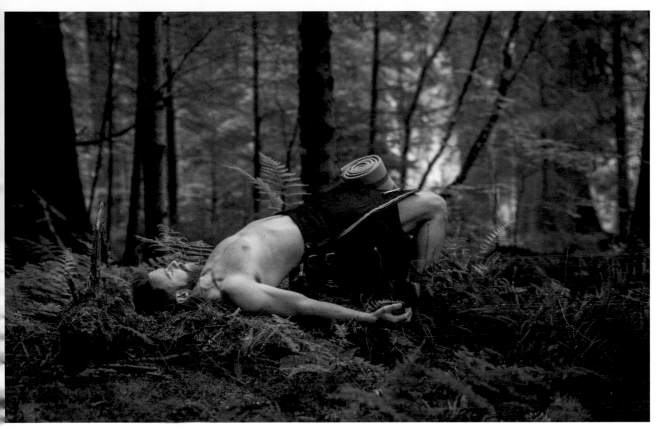

BRIDGE | 8–10 BREATHS

Place feet close to hips, hip-width apart, palms facing up and
about 1 foot away from hips. Neck stays still. Exhale, tuck the
tail bone and lift the pelvis. Connect to the strength in your legs.

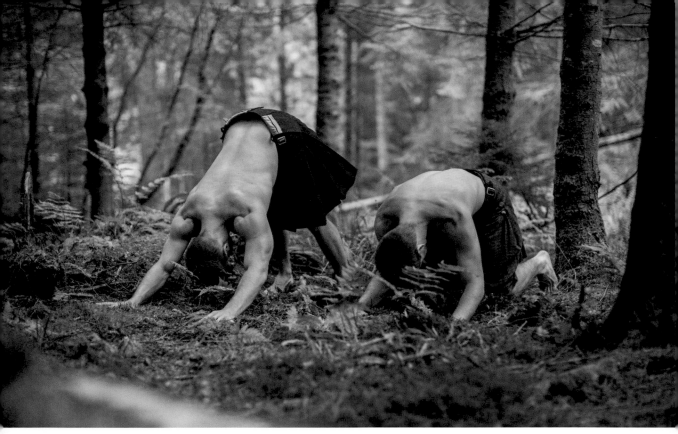

TURBO DOG | 10 BREATHS

From all fours, walk hands forwards 6 inches and bend the elbows. Inhale to round the upper back. Exhale, flex the chest, squeezing the upper arms towards each other, and lift the knees.

OPTION: *Try a Turbo Puppy, keeping your knees down to protect the wrists and shoulders.*

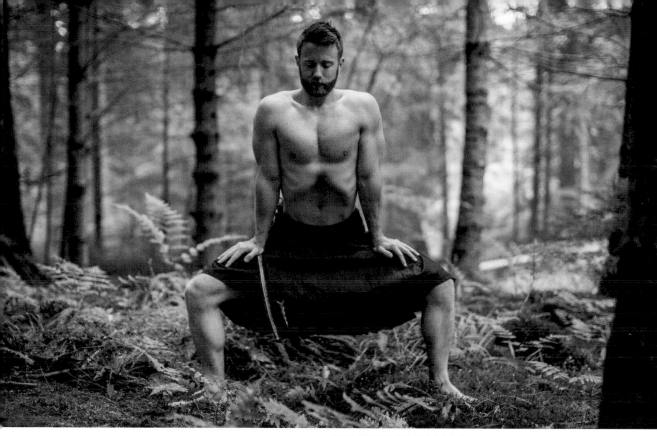

UDDIYANA IN HORSE | 4 ROUNDS

Stand with your legs 3 feet apart and your feet turned out
45 degrees. Bend the legs and brace your hands on thighs.
Exhale completely and hold. Scoop ribs up away from legs.
Hold for a count of ten. Then relax the belly and inhale.

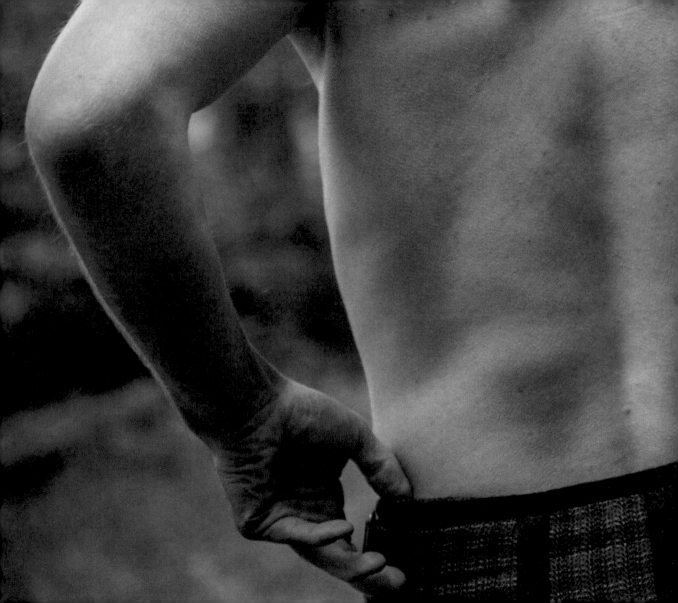

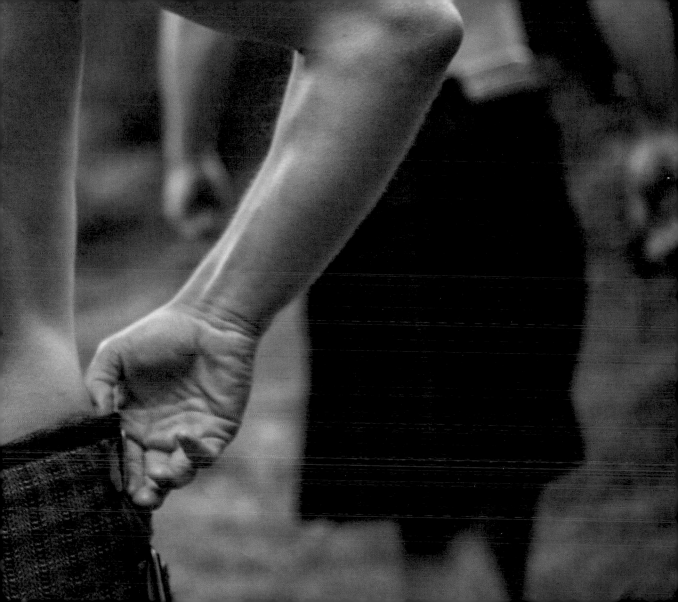

SUN SALUTATION | 4 ROUNDS

Standing, Arms Up, Forward Bend, Lunge, Plank, Low
Cobra, Downward-facing Dog, Lunge, Forward Bend,
Arms Up, Standing.

Inhale, Arms Up.

Exhale, Forward Bend.

Inhale, step right foot back into Lunge.

Exhale, take left foot back into Plank. Lower to ground.

Inhale, Low Cobra.

Exhale, Downward-facing Dog.

Inhale, step right foot forward into Lunge.

Exhale, bring left foot to meet right. Forward Bend.

Inhale, Arms Up.

Exhale, hands to chest.

(Alternate the legs in Lunge pose for each round.)

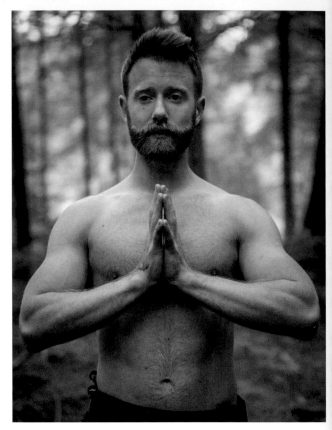

STANDING

Tuck the tail bone down and feel your active feet.

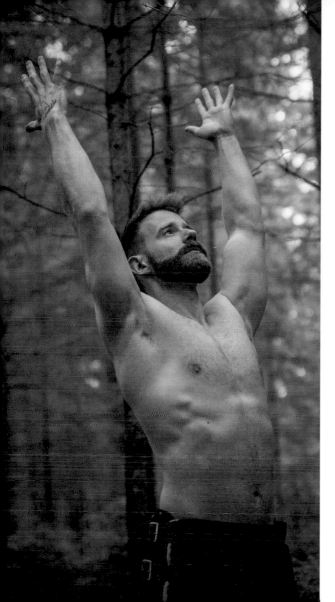

ARMS UP

Inhale to reach arms up while engaging through your thighs.

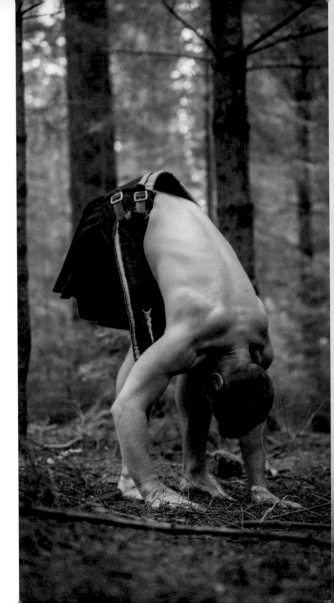

FORWARD BEND

Exhale to bend forward with knees bent.

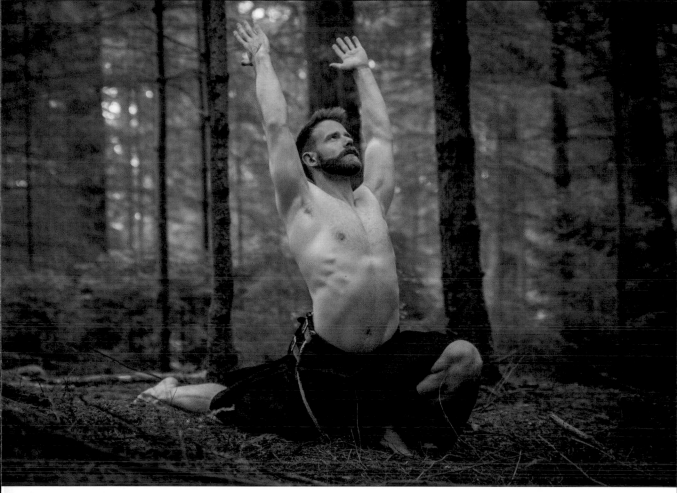

LUNGE

Inhale to Lunge pose, arms up.

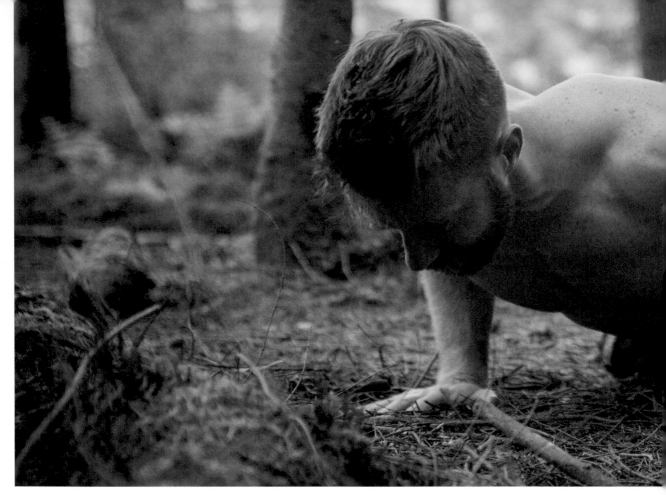

PLANK

Exhale to Plank pose. Lower to the ground.

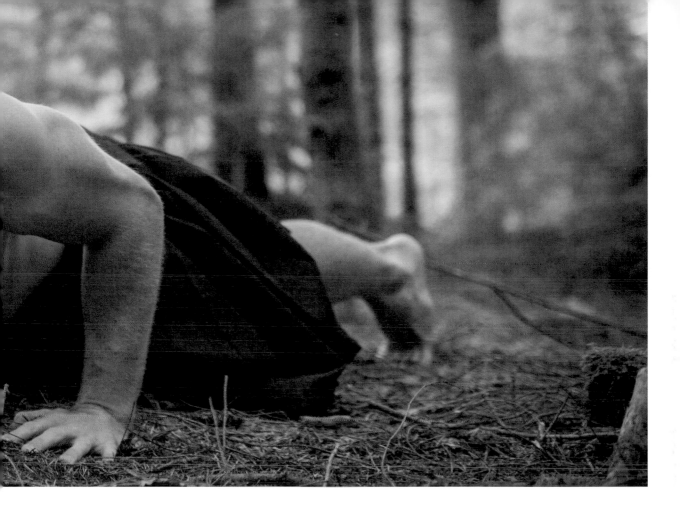

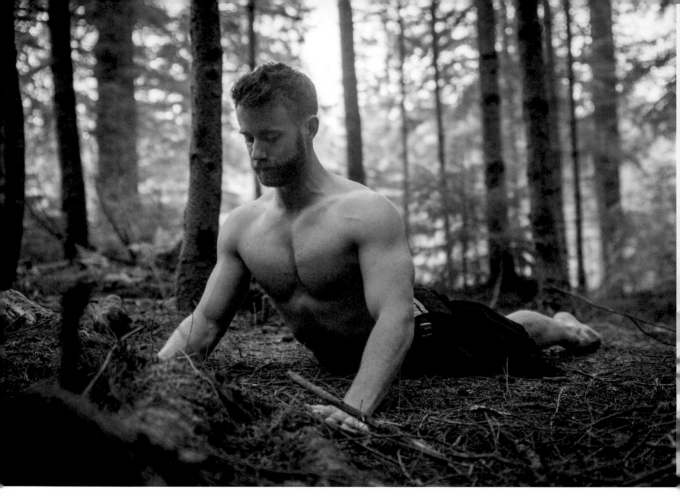

LOW COBRA

Inhale to Low Cobra pose. Pull the chest forwards.

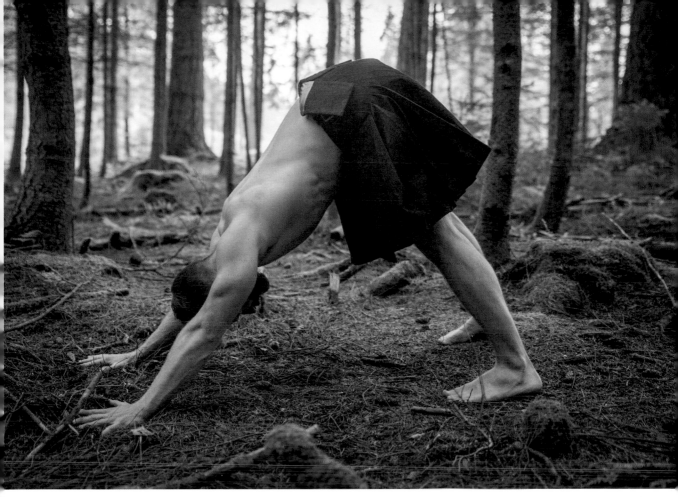

DOWNWARD-FACING DOG

Exhale to Downward-facing Dog pose. Lift your knees up.

OPTION: *Do Turbo Dog (see page 122) instead to build strength.*

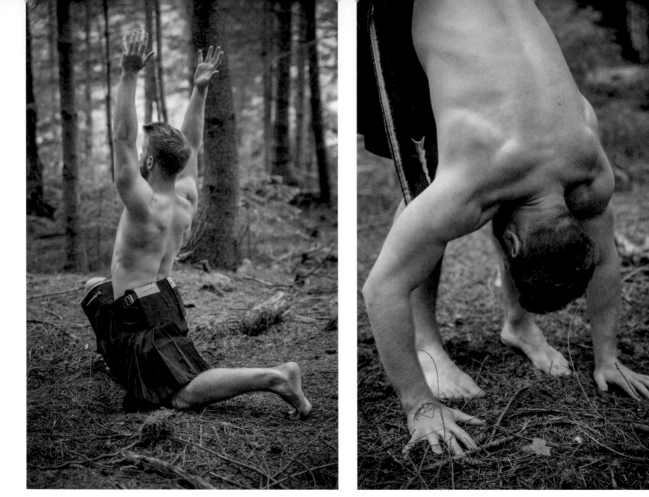

LUNGE

Inhale to Lunge pose, arms up.

FORWARD BEND

Exhale to bend forward, knees bent.

134

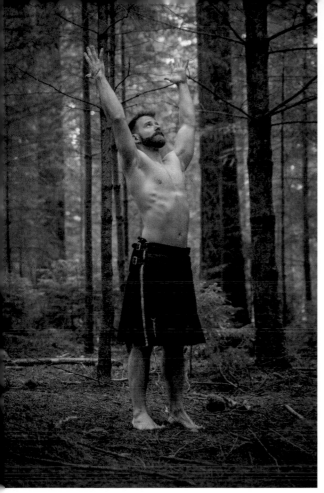

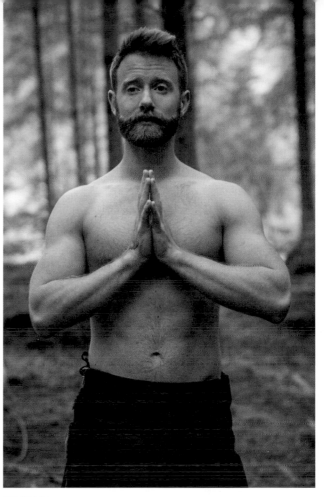

ARMS UP

Inhale to reach up.

STANDING

Exhale, hands to chest.

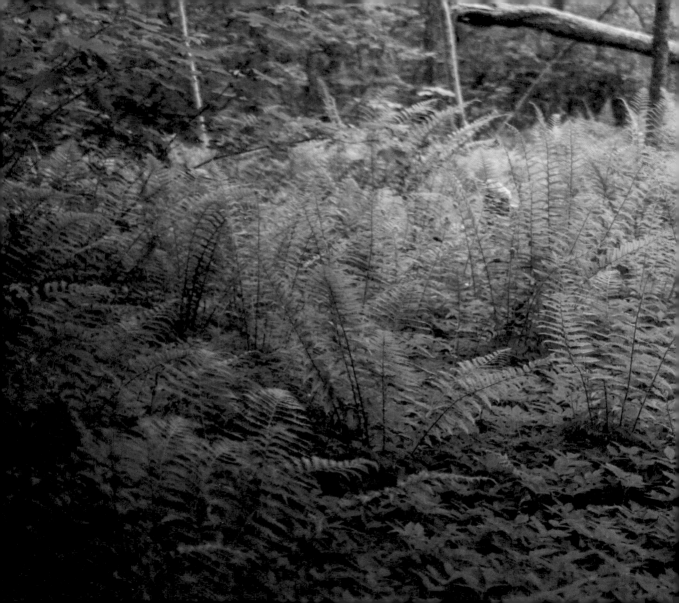

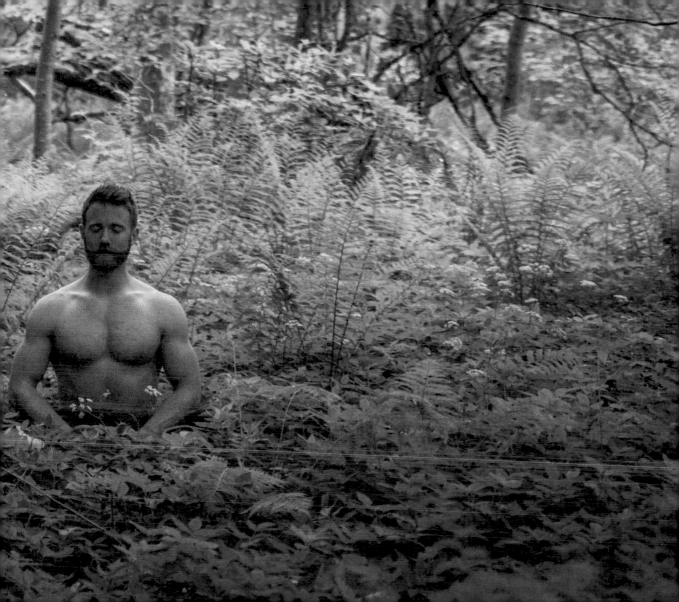

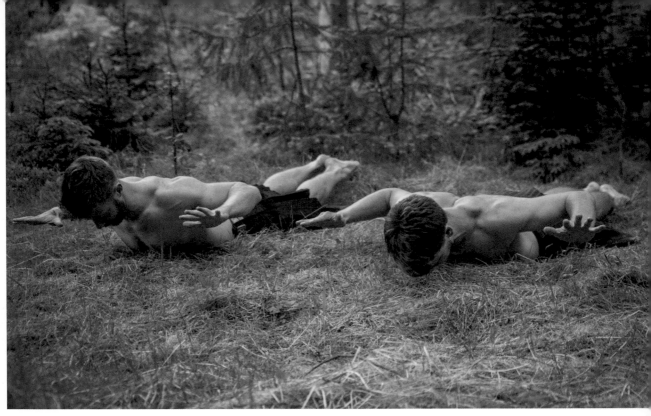

BOAT SHRUGS | 5 ROUNDS

Lying down, place hands in line with head. Inhale to lift your chest and legs.

Exhale, squeeze shoulder blades together and reach through the legs. Inhale to relax shoulder blades, keeping the chest and legs lifted. Stay up throughout all the rounds.

OPTION: *Feet can stay on the ground to keep the pressure off the lower back.*

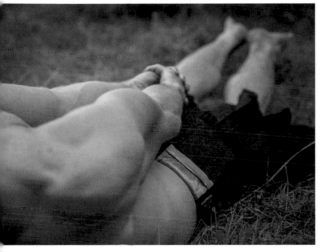

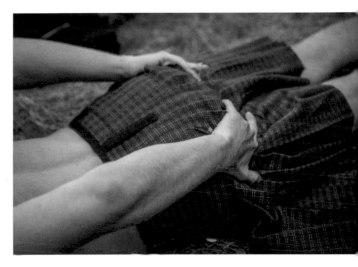

BOAT | 5 BREATHS

Clasp your hands at your lower back. Inhale to lift the chest and the legs. Exhale, draw your shoulder blades towards each other and tuck your tail bone.

OPTION: *Grab your sit bones and feel the lower buttock muscles engaging. Feet stay on the ground.*

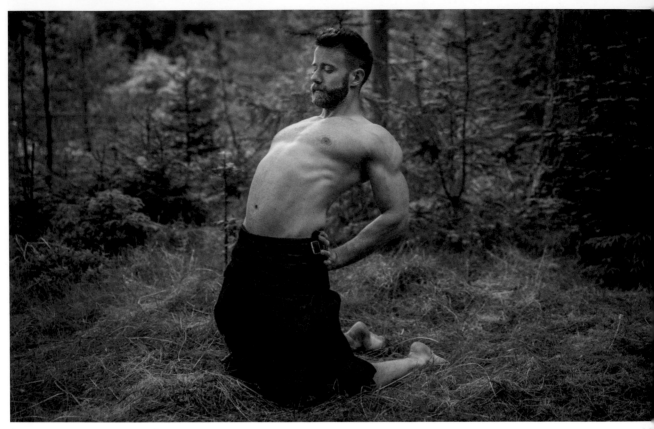

CAMEL HANDS ON HIPS | 8 BREATHS

Kneeling down, place hands on the pelvis, thumbs touching.

Exhale, tuck the tail bone down. Inhale to telescope the ribs up.

Chin rests forwards. Keep your hips above your knees.

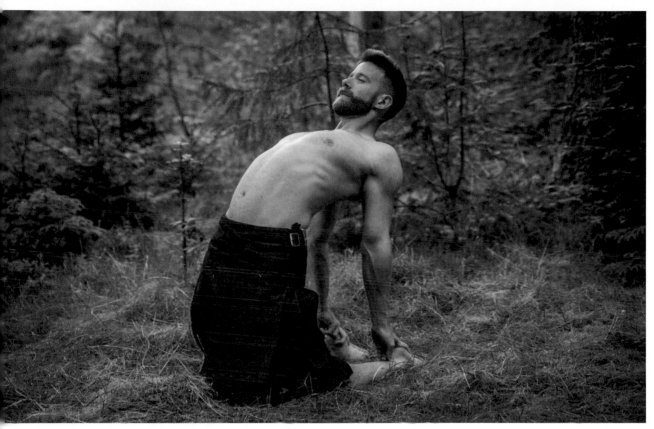

CAMEL HANDS ON HEELS | 8 BREATHS

From Camel Hands on Hips, if comfortable to do, reach hands towards the heels. If this is too much, repeat the previous pose.

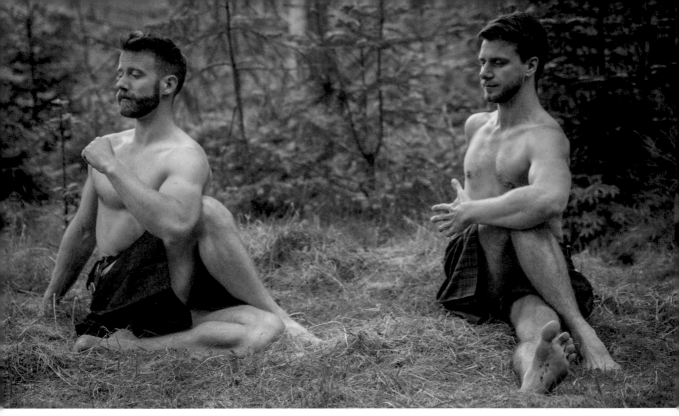

CLASSICAL TWIST | 5 BREATHS

Cross right leg over the bent left leg. Either hold the right shin
with left forearm or cross the left elbow outside the right leg.
Right hand supports behind. Inhale to lift the ribs. Exhale to
twist right, chin in line with chest. Repeat on the other side.

OPTION: *Work with the bottom leg straight if bending the leg
is making the hips lopsided.*

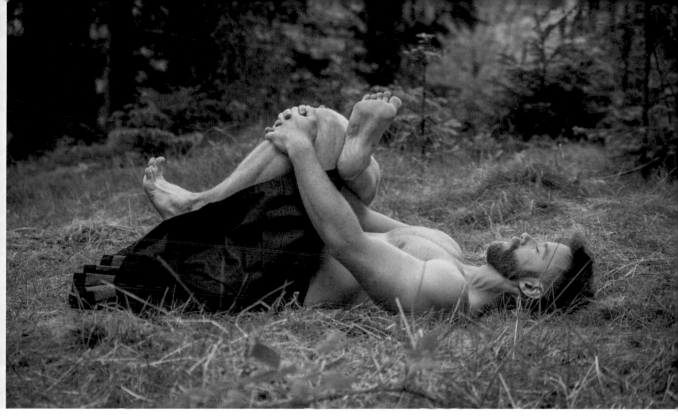

BACK RELEASE | 8 BREATHS PER SIDE

Cross right ankle over the left knee. Exhale to bring the legs
closer to the chest and reach the right arm through the gap.
Clasp your hands to hold the left thigh. Press your lower back
into the mat. Repeat on the other side.

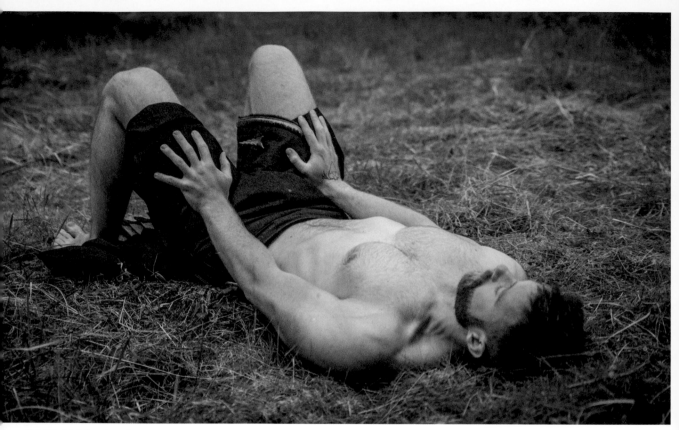

BACK TRACTION | 5 BREATHS

Plant the feet hip-distance apart. Brace the hands on the
thighs and scoop the ribs away from the pelvis. Combine
this with a strong pulling in of the belly on each exhale.

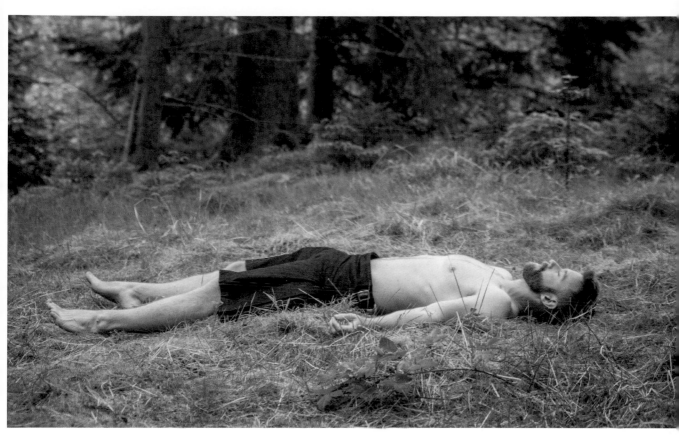

SAVASANA

Relax completely.

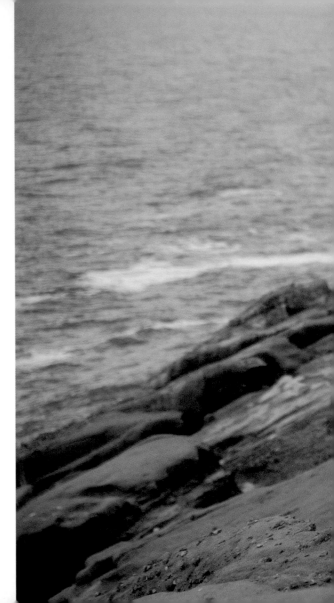

WALKING MEDITATION

Choose somewhere that you are familiar with to walk to and make sure you won't be interrupted by your mobile ringing. Decide on a route or destination. Begin a steady walking pace and start inhaling for four steps and exhaling for six. Repeat this and stay connected to how your body and mind react to working in this way.

As you become more proficient at the breathing exercises, begin to increase the count by one but always keeping the exhale for two steps longer than the inhale.

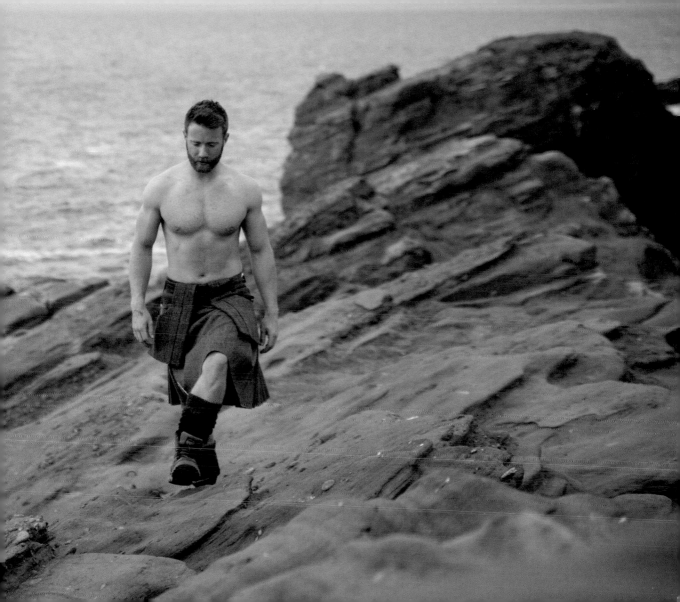

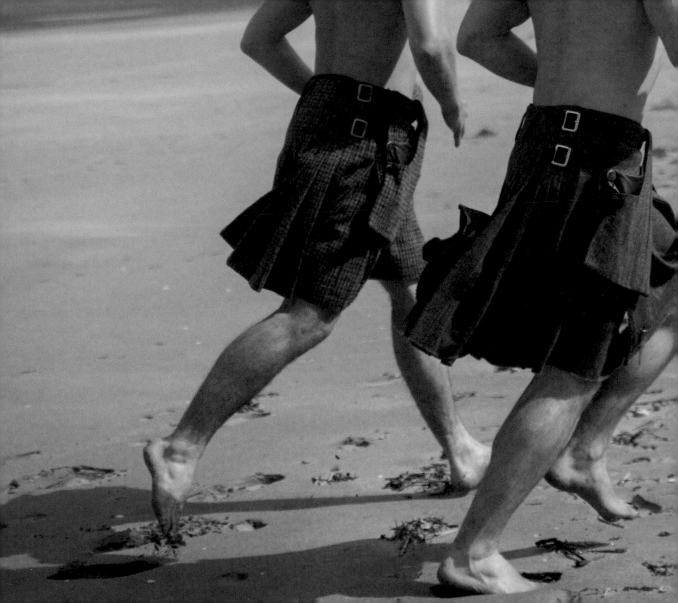

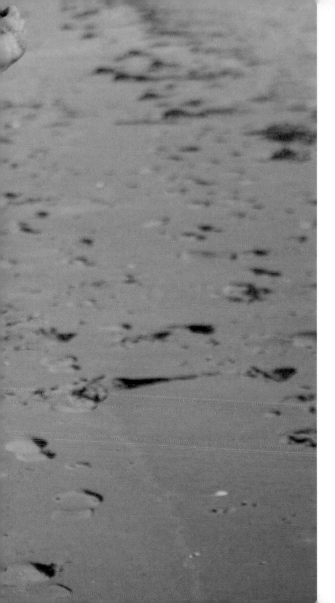

DOUBLE POSES

One great thing about a yoga practice is sharing it with another person. You keep each other going, motivating and assisting each other. And you can enjoy maintaining the focus with ease when someone else is there practising with you. This section introduces you to poses you can easily do together at home!

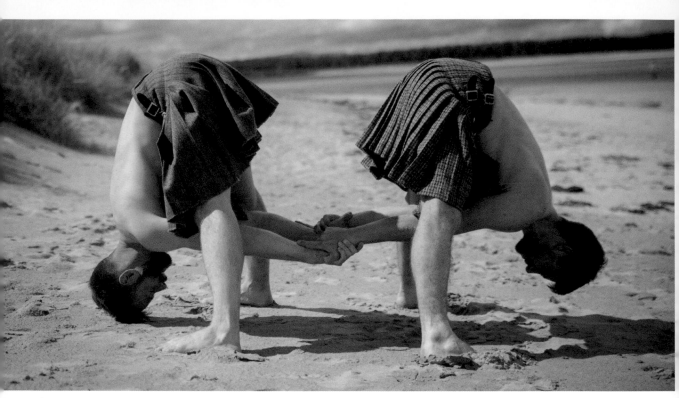

DOUBLE STRADDLE

Stand facing away from each other about 2 feet apart. Have the feet set wider than your shoulders and parallel. Fold from your hips, legs bent and reach for each other's hands. Brace at the wrists for a firm grip, and lean away from each other to feel the counterbalance and increase the stretch.

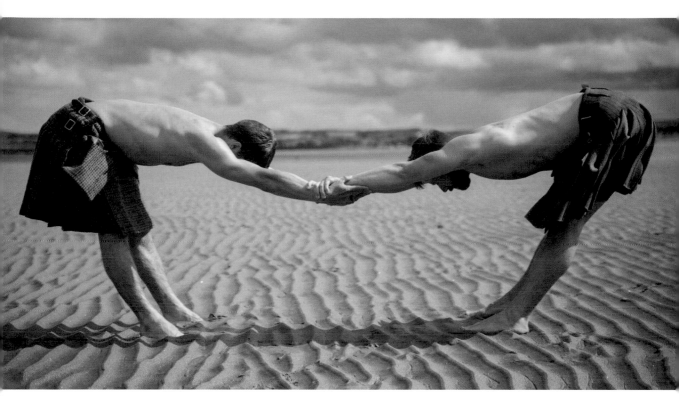

SUSPENSION BRIDGE

From standing, hold your partner's wrists. Bend the knees and
fold forwards until chests are parallel to the ground. Gradually
straighten the legs and lean away from each other. Enjoy the
stretch in the lower back.

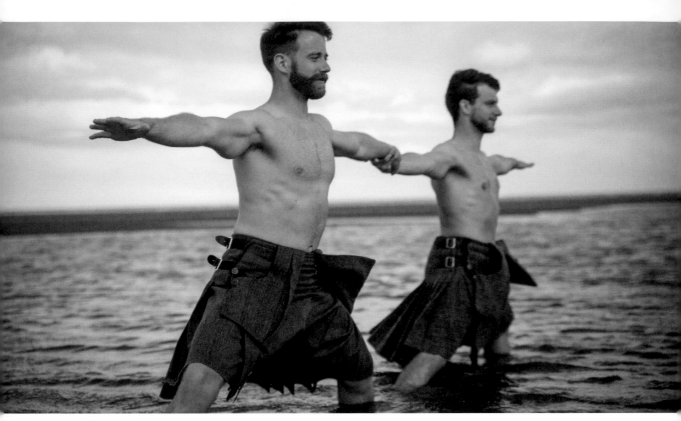

DOUBLE WARRIOR

Stand in Warrior II (see page 102) with your back foot against your partner's. Brace at the wrists and lean into the counterbalance.

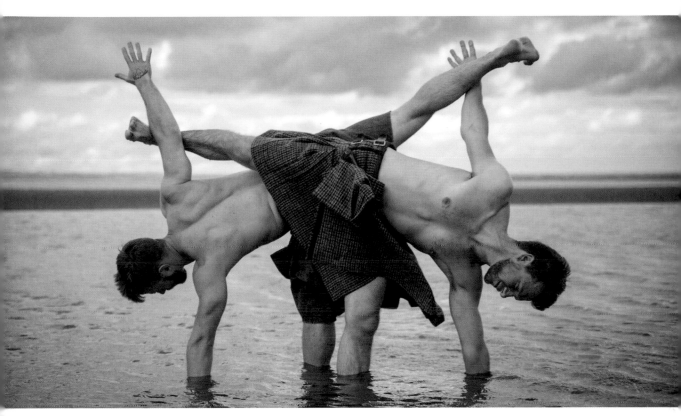

TWIN MOON

Stand back to back in Warrior II with the left leg bent. Extend the left arm forward and onto the ground in front of your foot, shifting your weight onto your left side. Lift the right leg, then hook your right arm around your partner's lifted leg and feel the challenging balance.

FAQs

HOW DO I FIND A YOGA TEACHER?

Searching online for teachers can be really tricky, especially if you live in a rural area. Some teachers may only run a small class in a community centre and not have the information on a website. I always prefer to work with recommendations, so ask your friends whom they go to or if they know of anyone. Take the time to look in community centres or libraries for information about locally run classes.

WHAT ABOUT FORREST YOGA, WHERE CAN I LOOK?

This is a much more focused search as Forrest Yoga teachers are less common. You can find information about registered teachers at www.forrestyoga.com and use the search function for your area. Some teachers may call it a Forrest-inspired class; that works too.

I AM NOT FLEXIBLE, CAN I DO YOGA?

Saying you aren't flexible enough is like saying you are too dirty to wash! Flexibility is not a prerequisite of yoga but yoga can certainly help you develop body awareness, and increase your flexibility and strength to do some of the more advanced poses. Remember, you are not in a rush to get flexible, so take your time and be patient.

HOW OFTEN SHOULD I PRACTISE?

You will feel the difference in your body from doing yoga once a week. Set yourself a realistic goal. Twenty minutes a few times a week will do more for you than one binge session a week. I see a lot of people set out with the intention of doing 90 minutes every day and that might happen initially, but it is rarely maintained. Start small.

IS THERE AN OPTIMUM TIME OF DAY TO PRACTISE?

My personal preference is in the afternoon as my body is more willing to move, but doing yoga in the morning sets me up for the day ahead and allows me to sort my head out. Explore practising at different times and see what works best for you.

I HAVE AN INJURY, CAN I DO YOGA?

Of course. I recommend working with a teacher who has experience with injuries. One of the great things about Forrest Yoga is its ability to be adapted to provide modifications if a person has an injury. Build up a relationship with your teacher and explore working with the injury. If you aren't working with a teacher, remember that pain is an indication that something has to change. Stay out of the pain-giving area and explore the poses with compassion for that injured part. The Strength and Power sequences have some options to modify the poses too.

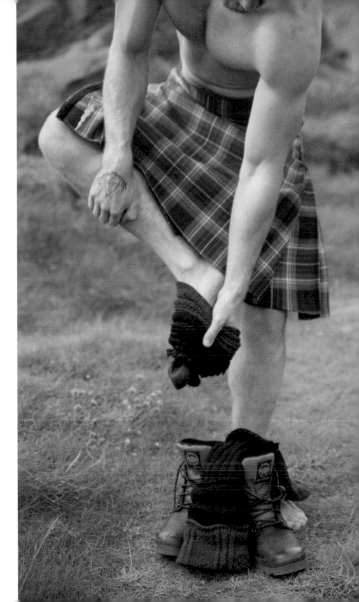

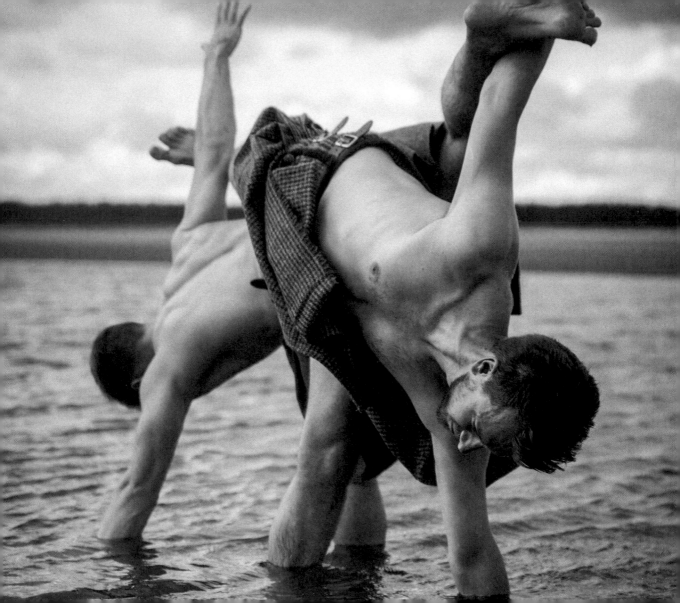

I DON'T HAVE A FAMILY NAME THAT HAS A TARTAN, WHICH ONES CAN I WEAR?

It is advised that you shouldn't wear a family tartan if you have no connection to the name just because you like the Sett (pattern) or the colours. There are tartans that are deemed 'public', meaning anyone can wear them. These range from districts (like my Heartland blue and green kilt) to place names and fashion and corporate tartans.

However, kilts do not need to be made in tartan. Remember that a kilt is a garment and tartan is a fabric! 21st Century Kilts use contemporary materials, ranging from Savile Row suiting, Harris Tweed, denims and tweeds sourced from all over the UK.

HOW DO YOU WEAR A KILT THAT IS NOT FOR A FORMAL OCCASION?

Kilts are the true alternative for men instead of trousers. You are able to dress down even a tartan kilt. By wearing boots and scrunching socks down it gives a less formal feel. I like to dress mine down with a T-shirt or a casual shirt.

I AM NOT SCOTTISH AND DO NOT HAVE SCOTTISH HERITAGE. CAN I WEAR A KILT?

The form of the kilt dates back to ancient Egyptian, Greek and Roman times. All cultures throughout the world have skirt-type garments for men as part of their history. The definition of a 'kilt' dates back to the Danish '*kilte*', meaning 'to tuck up', and Old Norse '*kjalta*', meaning 'to fold'. With this long heritage, it is often associated with Scotland but it isn't restricted to Scottish heritage.

The original kilt was a big wrap of material called a Breacan or the Great Kilt, which was wrapped across the body. The kilts that I wear are made for everyday wear and for anyone in the world to wear as an alternative to trousers. They sit a little lower than the traditional kilt and are fitted with pockets specific to 21st Century Kilts.

WHAT'S UNDER YOUR KILT?

Catch me on a windy day and you'll find out! Or you could always turn to the last page of the book …

INDEX

ACKNOWLEDGEMENTS

Many people have contributed to my yoga practice and have stood by me through challenging times.

I am grateful to the students that have joined me on the mat over the last few years who, with ongoing interaction, have opened up to me, shared their stories and, in turn, have fueled my drive to teach.

My most respected teacher, Ana Forrest, to whom I owe a debt of gratitude, not only for sharing with me her wisdom and practices to heal others, but for sending me on a path towards healing myself.

Huge thanks to the team at Hodder & Stoughton for putting this book together and to Andrew Smith for his fantastic design. Being able to shoot the book in some of my favourite places was incredible and the shots from Simon Buxton speak for themselves.

Thanks to Joel Wilson, my dear friend and fellow yoga teacher, for his patience and play in the creation of the book and sequences.

Thanks to the team at BBC The Social for the opportunity to create content with a Scottish voice and for all the support during some challenging times.

To my family, my gratitude for putting up with endless messages and photos of my backside!

Finally, a big thank you to Ian Alexander, whose unwavering support makes a lot of what I do possible.

RESOURCES

21ST CENTURY KILTS, EDINBURGH
21stcenturykilts.com
Kilt supplier, ships internationally

YOGA WEBSITES
www.finlay-wilson.com
www.yoga.heartspacedundee.co.uk
www.mat2mat.com/channels/finlay
www.youtube.com/user/Finlay0901
www.forrestyoga.com

SCOTTISH TOURIST BOARD
www.visitscotland.com

BBC THE SOCIAL
www.bbcthesocial.co.uk

LOCATIONS
Arbroath, Glen Coe, the Hermitage, Loch Earn and St Andrews

Publisher **LIZ GOUGH**
Project Editor **NATALIE BRADLEY**
Design and Art Direction **ANDREW SMITH**
Photography **SIMON BUXTON**
Props **21ST CENTURY KILTS**
Model **JOEL WILSON**
Senior Designer **SARAH CHRISTIE**
Production Manager **CLAUDETTE MORRIS**

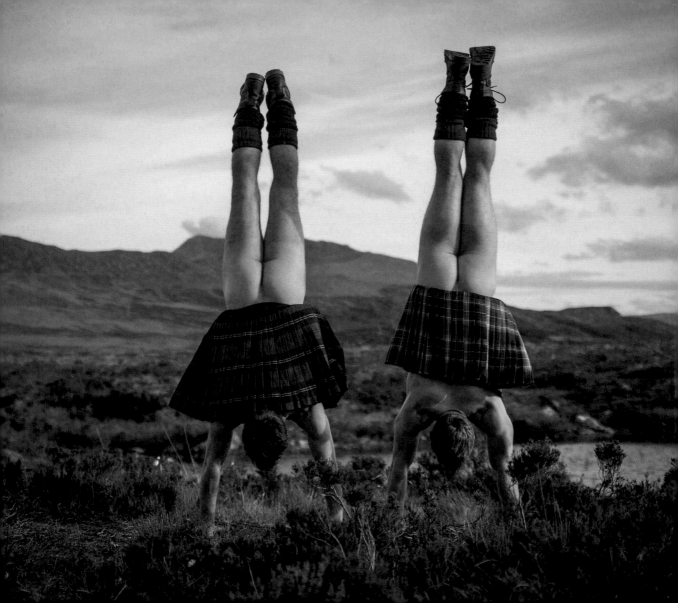